CONTENTS

SO-DMQ-853

084671

ACKNOWLEDGMENTS

I am grateful:

To my husband Bill, for his continued support, positive encouragement, and love.

To our daughter Juli and son Matt, for loving me through the kitchen experiments and lifestyle changes.

To my precious mother, who taught me to love and care for others by her example.

To Dorothy Galde, who edited the book, advised me, and believed in me.

To Susanne Galloway, who willingly did research and stayed by my side through it all.

To my faithful secretary, Eloise Funk, who made my workload easier.

To those in the fields of medicine, nutrition, and research who led seminars, taught classes, and wrote books to expand my horizons and teach me how to get well.

To Kin Millen, who believed in my ideas and encouraged me as a writer.

To the many friends, clients, and relatives who pushed me by asking when the book would be published.

To Barbara Spangler for her help in typing this manuscript.

To Jim Ruark, my editor at Zondervan, for mastering the details to get this book into print.

To Carol Holquist, at Zondervan, for always being there when I needed her.

I am also grateful for the publishers' permission to quote from the following works:

James W. Anderson, M.D., *Diabetes* (New York: Arco Publishing, 1981).

John D. Kirschmann, *Nutrition Almanac,* rev. ed. (New York: McGraw-Hill Book Company, 1975.

BLUEPRINT
FOR HEALTH

HOW DOES YOUR NUTRITION STACK UP?

MARY ANN HOWARD, R.N.

PYRANEE
BOOKS

Zondervan Publishing House
Grand Rapids, Michigan

Blueprint for Health:
How Does Your Nutrition Stack Up?

This is a Pyranee Book
Published by the Zondervan Publishing House
1415 Lake Drive, S.E., Grand Rapids, Michigan 49506

The information in this book is purely for educational purposes. The general nutrition guidelines offered toward physical and mental well-being do not constitute the diagnosis or treatment of disease. The reader is advised to consult his or her personal physician for specific application of dietary principles to best fit individual needs and remedy specific ailments.

Library of Congress Cataloging in Publication Data

Howard, Mary Ann.
    Blueprint for health.

    "Pyranee books."
    Bibliography: p.
    Includes index.
    1. Nutrition. 2. Health. I. Title.
RA784.H64   1985   613.2   85-22557
ISBN 0-310-42151-9

Unless otherwise indicated, the Scripture text used is the *New American Standard Bible,* copyright © 1960, 1962, 1963, 1968, 1971, 1972 by the Lockman Foundation, La Habra, California.

Edited by Carol Uridil and James E. Ruark
Designed by Ann Cherryman

Printed in the United States of America

    86   87   88   89   89   90   /   10   9   8   7   6   5   4   3   2

PREFACE

When I was in nursing school in the fifties, the study of nutrition was practically nonexistent.

My first encounter with poor health came after I became a registered nurse. I began to suspect that stress and improper eating habits might have contributed to my failing health. So in 1956 I started a search for clues to my health problems, and since then I have gained much knowledge and found many pieces to the puzzle of finding and maintaining good health.

A poor diet often contributes to illness. Doughnuts, coffee, fried meat, french-fried potatoes, pie à la mode, candy bars, hot dogs with mustard, ice cream, sweetened cola drinks, synthetic vitamins and chemicals added to food, and aspirin to alleviate discomfort can't make for good health. Since we are what we eat and assimilate, we should make our choices wisely.

We are currently in a drug age in America in which the solution for every illness seems to be a multitude of chemical pills. These pills are seldom harmless, and they are often lethal. Many drugs only mask the symptoms of the illnesses being treated and may cause serious side effects that are even worse than the original disease. Although drugs are necessary, they can be abused.

My aim is to help you benefit from my mistakes. By sharing my successful do-it-yourself program, I hope to motivate you to take positive steps toward better health. I want to encourage you, give you hope, and help you set goals toward constructive change that may result in more vibrant health.

This book is not an attempt to give you answers to your medical problems; the diagnosis and treatment of disease is your physician's responsibility. Consult him about specific ailments; he is trained and qualified to assist you. The guidelines set forth in these pages are to teach you *health maintenance* and help you *prevent disease*.

The case histories presented are from my office files. Names have been changed to protect the privacy of my counselees.

1   WHERE DID I GO WRONG?

As I walked toward the platform to receive my diploma, I was accompanied by gnawing stomach pains and fatigue. It was August 1952, and my dream was coming true: I was graduating from Ball Memorial Hospital School of Nursing in Muncie, Indiana. And I was determined to be the best registered nurse ever to graduate from there. My five-foot-three-inch frame looked healthy, but my skin was pale, and I weighed only a hundred pounds. *If only those gnawing stomach pains would leave me alone, . . .* I thought.

Those years in nurses' training kept me extremely busy. The classes were difficult and required long hours of study. I was on a scholarship and wanted to earn good grades. The work in the hospital was exciting but tiring because of the constant life-and-death situations that faced us. My fiancé would drive sixty miles from Indianapolis to see me every free weekend. I was extra busy as president of the senior class. With all this going on, there was little time to eat, and I skipped many meals. When hunger pangs came, I snacked on candy, ice cream, cake, cola drinks, salty nuts, pretzels, and potato chips.

When I did sit down to eat, I ate large quantities of beef, pork, potatoes, and bread, and my food was seldom touched until I sprinkled it with a heavy layer of salt. The other foods I relished were sour cream, whipped cream, butter, fat meat, gravies, and sauces. Vegetables and fruits didn't appeal to me, and I thought water was strictly for bathing.

Sleep was neglected to accomplish my goal of becoming a registered nurse. While night duty robbed me of sleep, daytime classes and activities kept me from getting the rest I needed.

Three weeks before graduation and my twenty-first birthday, the doctor said the gnawing pains in my stomach were caused by a duodenal ulcer. I had no time for this interference because I was also planning my wedding.

One month after graduation on September 28, 1952, I married Bill, the love of my life. I passed the State Nursing Board Exam and was employed as a registered nurse in a hospital, but before three months had passed, my career was suddenly shelved. After a week of unbearable chest pain, I suddenly began to gasp for breath. My left lung had collapsed. Unable to diagnose the cause, my doctor gave me tuberculosis drugs as a precautionary measure, but eighteen months after good health had been restored, my right lung collapsed. A fluid culture revealed that tuberculosis bacilli were alive and active. One year of complete bed rest and strong tuberculosis drugs eventually eliminated the disease.

Throughout my illness I was told to eat anything I wanted, just as long as I ate three meals a day. As you might guess, my diet included all my favorite foods—high in fat, high in salt, and high in sugar.

Bill and I had been married only three months when I first became sick, and my humorous husband would laughingly exclaim, "When you get a car that's a lemon, you simply trade it in; but when you get a wife that's a lemon, you're stuck with her." Proverbs 17:22 KJV states, "A merry heart doeth good like a medicine: but a broken spirit drieth the bones." We tried to keep a sense of humor and find things to laugh about when times were difficult.

Six years later my hopes of bearing children were shattered when a ruptured tubal pregnancy nearly ended my life. I was never able to get pregnant after that. When migraine headaches and depression became a way of life, the prescribed treatment was tranquilizers, pain pills, mood elevators, and sleeping pills. After that regime was established, an eye hemorrhage developed, which caused temporary loss of sight in my right eye. No diagnosis could be made. The advice I received was to simply live with the problem and forget it happened.

Two years later diabetes was diagnosed, and for the first time I was told to eliminate sugar from my diet.

The crowning blow came when intermittent attacks of joint pain started. As these progressed my joints became stiff, swollen, and excruciatingly painful. My physician said, "I can find no apparent cause, but it must be rheumatoid arthritis." The arthritis drugs caused side effects and had to be discontinued. My doctor said, "Take three aspirin every three hours and learn to live with it." But when I did this, my ulcer flared up again.

In desperation Bill and I cried out: "O God, help us." A doctor friend suggested we move to a warmer climate so I would be more comfortable during the cold winter months. All other doors seemed to have been closed to us. What were we to do?

In April 1966 we left our family and lifelong friends behind and moved to Phoenix, Arizona. Our two beautiful adopted children were five and six. Although we didn't know a soul in Phoenix, the hot, dry air of this lovely desert land soothed my aching body. But even there, my poor health prevented me from working as a nurse—it was difficult enough just taking care of the children.

Shortly after our move, we found a church to meet our spiritual needs. We attended regularly and studied the Bible enthusiastically. The church members helped and encouraged us, and we made many new friends. Our faith in God grew, and our personal relationship with Jesus Christ developed.

Our friends showed concern about my health problems and started making suggestions: one suggested a diet change; another an exercise program; and others recommended books.

My initial reason for becoming a registered nurse was to help sick people, but when I ended up as sick as most of my patients, I began to search for answers to my health problems. As I studied books on food, its nutrients, and diet as it relates to disease, biochemistry, exercise programs, and health, a new world unfolded.

I decided to take a refresher course in nursing, after which I worked for a short time in a hospital. Several patients under my care had the same diseases I had battled. When I saw that they were being given many drugs and were still as chronically ill as I was, I became frustrated and realized I could no longer administer doubtful drugs to sick people. Then a thought struck me, "Ye have not, because ye ask not" (James 4:2 KJV). So I asked God's direction. Since my interest was being focused toward helping people stay well and teaching sick people to make lifestyle and diet changes to improve their health, I quit my job and began searching for answers to some of these problems.

I enrolled in classes to study biochemistry and nutrition and attended seminars on diet and disease. My nursing background enabled me to understand the functions of the human body as they related to these subjects. I gained a new understanding of the basic needs of the body's cells. God designed the human body, and he made food and its nutrients to fit into the cells and energize them. While I accompanied my husband on business trips to Europe, I sought out medical doctors working in nutrition and degenerative disease, and I corresponded with others who were writing books on these subjects. My own body became the testing ground for my new discoveries. Shortly after I began my experimental self-help program, another thought hit me: Could I have abused my body unknowingly?

There are basic divine rules that need to be obeyed—had I broken some of them? God's way, not our way, is always best. I had tried it my way, and it hadn't worked. Proverbs 1:5 admonishes, "A wise man will hear and increase in learning, and a man of understanding will acquire wise counsel" (NASB). I asked God for wisdom in working out a new pattern for my life.

In the chapters that follow I explain some changes in my lifestyle that I believe have greatly contributed to my improved health. I have often said, "I was one of the sickest young women in our town, but I am going to be one of the healthiest *older* women in town."

For a number of years I have been privileged to counsel people privately in the areas of diet change, exercise, and ways to deal with stress, and I have set up nutrition programs for people of all ages. It has been rewarding to see many of them regain their health. Numerous others improved their health when they made the effort to follow the guidelines I gave them. Often nothing more was required than an awareness of and a return to the basic things God designed for their bodies.

Millions of people are ruining their bodies by giving in to their appetites. It is sad. If the body doesn't have what it needs to function, it won't. Dietary excesses, as well as deficiencies lead to trouble.

2 PREVENTION—THE NAME OF THE GAME

Every day in my nutritional-counseling office, I hear a common complaint: "I don't feel well. I'm so tired." I hear this from young and old alike and know that the kind of exhaustion they are talking about is simply not eliminated by rest.

Often when I check the medical history of a patient, I find that her doctor, after a physical examination, has pronounced her perfectly healthy. This puzzles me. A medical book in my library lists several potential organic causes for fatigue, chronic exhaustion, and lethargy. They are chronic infections, anemia, endocrine and metabolic disorders, chronic poisoning, habitual use of depressants or sedative drugs, malignancy, connective-tissue disease, and any debilitating illness.[1] With all these possible causes, why is fatigue not diagnosed and treated more often?

Roberta is a thirty-one-year-old wife and mother who, when I first met her, was taking medication for a rapid heartbeat (tachycardia). She complained of water retention in her hands and feet, headaches, digestive problems, and extreme fatigue. Her typical daily diet consisted of toast and jelly for breakfast; a bologna sandwich, cheese, crackers, and ice cream for lunch; and a TV dinner, meat, or chicken for her evening meal. For snacks she would eat ice cream with chocolate syrup or occasionally fruit.

In answer to my question about exercise, she said, "I don't exercise, though I know I would feel better if I did." Then I asked, "How much water do you drink each day?" She responded, "Hardly any. I drink mostly coffee, iced tea, and soft drinks." When I asked her how long she had eaten that way, she answered, "Since college my diet has been poor. I ate mostly junk food throughout my college years. I craved sweets, and sometimes I would eat as many as ten candy bars a day."

So after I suggested she start an exercise program, she

signed up for an aerobic dance class that met five times a week at the local spa. I advised her to set up a body- and bowel-cleansing regime and suggested she drink six ounces of water eight times a day. Then we worked on diet changes; salt, sugar, fats, and caffeine were the four problem areas that needed the most attention.

She was to eat eggs or whole-grain cereals, whole-wheat toast, and fruit for breakfast. For lunch and dinner we planned a wide variety of raw vegetables in salads or lightly steamed. She would use vegetables in abundance. Fish, chicken, turkey, and occasionally beef, as well as low-fat dairy products were included, or a combination of beans and corn, or beans and rice, which are good sources of protein. Whole-grain breads and pasta could be added. Dessert should be fruit instead of cake, pie, and ice cream. Then I told her to go home and review her outlined program and pick out where she wanted to start. She would write those goals down and work on them before moving on.

I encouraged her to focus on only one area at a time because I have found that small changes are best; they require less discipline and are more apt to succeed. If changes are too drastic, people become overwhelmed and fail.

Two months later Roberta was pleased with her health improvement. Her stamina had increased, and often she was not tired at all. Her digestive problems had subsided, and her problem with water retention was gone. She exuded self-approval. She said, "My two boys have behaved much better these last two months. I don't know if it's because I'm feeling better or because I've cut out much of the sugar and junk food and substituted better meals and snacks for all of us. . . . I love the exercise program. My energy level is better when I exercise. On the two days I don't go to the spa, I'm lethargic."

We worked on additional changes for another year, and we saw many improvements. Her doctor, during one of her physical examinations, even stopped the medication for her rapid heartbeat. Then shortly after Christmas she called me and said, "During the holidays I felt bad again. I think I know why, too. I had pie, cake, candy, fatty foods, neglected my exercise, and in my mad rush, slipped back into the old habits. I need an appointment for a refresher course." And she also made an appointment for her husband to come in for his first nutritional consultation.

Think about your own lifestyle. Can you identify with Roberta? List any ways your lifestyle resembles hers.

1. _____

2. _____

3. _____

4. _____

5. _____

The Surgeon General reports, "Death from the major, acute, infectious diseases plummeted between 1900 and 1970. The proportion of mortality from chronic diseases, such as cancer, heart disease, and stroke, however, increased 250%. . . . The success of the first revolution means that the pattern of killing and disabling diseases has shifted drastically."[2] Although statistics like these often seem vague, we must realize that they are describing our families, our friends, and ourselves.

Since heart disease, cancer, and stroke are the major killers of our time, we need to fortify ourselves against them. To begin, we need to consider certain risk factors that relate to these diseases: age, lifestyle, diet, income, habits such as smoking or excessive use of alcohol, the places where we live or work that may be associated with a higher-than-average incidence of specific health problems. These risk factors are warning flags. Some are uncontrollable, such as age, sex, genetics, or diseases that are common in a family. But others are controllable. We have a choice in such matters as smoking, exercising, abusing alcoholic beverages, regularly brushing our teeth, maintaining a reasonable pattern of work and rest, and selecting the most appropriate diet.

In 1977 the chairman of the Senate Select Committee on Human Needs, George McGovern reported, "During this century, the composition of the average diet in the United States has changed radically. Foods containing complex carbohydrates and 'naturally occurring' sugars—fruit, vegetables and grain products—which were the mainstay of the diet, now play a minority role. During this time the consumption of fats and refined and processed sugars has risen to the point where these two macronutrients alone comprise at least 60% of total caloric intake, an increase of 20% since the early 1900's." It should also be noted that during this period the major killers of today surfaced. The report went on to say, "The overconsumption of the above foods plus salt and/or alcohol has been associated with the development of one or more of six to ten leading causes of death: heart disease, some cancers, stroke and hypertension, diabetes, arteriosclerosis and cirrhosis of the liver."[3]

When a friend of mine, who is a sugarholic, read this report, she remarked, "Well, we all have to die of something, don't we?"

On July 26, 1979, Joseph A. Califano, Jr., then Secretary of Health, Education and Welfare, said, "We are now coming to realize that victory over today's major killers—heart disease, cancer, stroke and others—must be achieved more by prevention than by cure."[4] He drew three conclusions, "1. We are killing ourselves by our own careless habits. 2. We are killing ourselves by carelessly polluting the environment. 3. We are killing ourselves by permitting harmful social conditions to persist—conditions like poverty, hunger and ignorance—which destroy health, especially for infants and children."[5]

But only 4 percent of the federal health dollar is spent for prevention-related activities. This means that 96 percent is spent on the treatment of disease. But improvement in our health will not be made primarily through the treatment, but through prevention. Prevention saves lives, improves the quality of life, and in the long run saves dollars.[6]

Thomas A. Edison was ahead of his time when he said, "The doctor of the future will give no medicine, but will interest his patients in the care of the human frame, in diet, and in the cause and prevention of disease."

Two case histories from my files illustrate this principle. Dave and Joan are married; they are both forty-five. When they first came to me for counseling, she had major complaints: she needed to lose weight; she suffered with headaches; and she was always tired in the early evening. Dave had slightly elevated blood pressure, and his energy level fell after lunch each day. By evening he was dragging. He also needed to lose weight. Their diets were the same: high-fat cheese was a mainstay; vegetables and fruits were almost nonexistent; meat was the focus of every meal; and eggs were eaten daily.

At my suggestion they started eating more whole grains and cereal instead of eggs in the morning. They added a variety of fresh vegetables and fruits to their meals and cut down on meat. Fish and chicken were used to add variety to their meat choices. They changed to low-fat dairy products and used fruit for dessert instead of sweets. Both of them cut down on table salt and began to drink more water. I asked them to start walking a mile a day, together, if possible. When they returned two months later to review their progress, Joan said, "My energy level has gone up so much that I now realize how tired I had been. We are really enjoying our walks, and we communicate much better during those times. It's just us—the kids aren't interrupting." She had lost six pounds, and her headaches had disappeared completely.

Dave remarked, "I hold on to my energy all day now and feel so much better. I sometimes exercise twice a day. In the morning with Joan and again after work." Then he surprised me by saying, "My doctor said my blood pressure was normal when I was there last week." He had not lost any weight, however. But on his next visit two months later, he had lost seven pounds.

Dave and Joan have five children and are beginning to ask questions about how to change their children's eating habits. It makes my work rewarding to realize how many people's health and lives may be affected by instructing one couple toward a better diet and lifestyle.

Are there any problems suggested by these case histories that you struggle with? List them.

1. _____

2. _____

3. _____

Do you think your diet and exercise habits have anything to do with your energy level, blood pressure, weight, and health problems? List how diet and exercise might help improve your own well-being.

1. _____

2. _____

3. _____

4. _____

Can you begin to see how we often create our own health problems? Just as there are physical laws of nature—like the law of gravity—there are laws connected with health and prevention of disease. If we defy the laws of nourishment, exercise, and rest for our bodies, there will be serious health consequences.

3 HOW DO WE APPROACH ILLNESS IN AMERICA?

When I try to imagine what a good doctor must be like, I think of Saint Luke, who was called the "beloved physician." Luke had all the qualities of an outstanding doctor, and his narratives reflect his interest in medical matters. He recounts the events surrounding two births—the birth of Christ and of John the Baptist. He was very interested in children and describes Jesus' childhood. Sensitive and understanding, he describes the inner thoughts of Jesus' mother, Mary. He often shows an uncommon interest in people and their needs. He had great respect for women and gives them a prominent place in his narratives. He was interested in people's living conditions, their poverty and wealth.[1] Had I lived in that part of the world at that time, I would have wanted Luke for my doctor.

Now, as then, we usually turn to doctors or other trained professionals when we are sick. But now there are other factors to consider that Luke's patients didn't have to be concerned about. Today we need to be very selective when choosing physicians, making sure they are qualified and have our best interest at heart. Doctors frequently prescribe drugs for certain conditions or suggest tests and X-rays, and after a diagnosis, they may prescribe more drugs or recommend surgery.

But the drugs themselves can be a problem. Dr. Robert S. Mendelsohn, a pediatrician in Chicago, argues, "Drugs are now being so over-prescribed that more illnesses are being caused by their side effects than are being cured. . . . Before accepting a prescription, demand that your doctor tell you about the medication, and if he refuses to, check the *Physician's Desk Reference* yourself before swallowing."[2] It is good advice.

According to the *New York Times,* "More than fifteen billion drug prescriptions are filled each year in the United States. Today every twenty-four to thirty-six hours, fifty to eighty percent of all adults in the United States swallow at least one medically prescribed drug."[3]

Because of my own experiences with prescription drugs, I am able to inform you on how to guard against their abuse. Sir Francis Bacon warned, "It is possible to cure the disease and kill the patient."

The following true accounts emphasize the possible dangers in the abuse of prescribed drugs.

Steve, the good-looking, forty-one-year-old Christian husband of Pat and father of two children, was scared. He sat on the edge of his bed in the psychiatric ward of St. Luke's Hospital in Phoenix, Arizona. His body shook as he begged the doctor to dismiss him.

Just two hours before, he had been admitted for withdrawal from Valium, a popular tranquilizer. He pleaded, "I've been summoned to appear in court tomorrow. I must be there."

"Why?" asked the psychiatrist.

"The district attorney notified me that I had written two bad checks. I don't remember doing it, but my wife says I did. My memory has many gaps. I have no money for a lawyer to represent me. I must appear or face a jail sentence."

"What started you on Valium?" the psychiatrist asked?

"Five years ago, I developed intense pain in my lower back. I went to an orthopedic surgeon. He gave me Darvon for pain and Valium to relax the muscle spasms. The drugs helped me cope with the problem. I felt wrapped in a protective cloud. They prevented anxious thoughts from crowding in on me. Three years ago I had a life-threatening heart attack and couldn't work. As the pressure built and bills stacked up, I became depressed."

"What happened then?" asked the psychiatrist.

"I took more Valium and Darvon to give me tranquillity. Soon I was getting refills every two weeks. Yesterday the pharmacy refused to refill my prescription. I had no more pills. Last evening, trembling all over, fear gripped me. I panicked. Filled with anxiety, my wife called you. I can't believe I'm here."

Steve, like many others, didn't plan to become an addict. He had never taken street drugs—only drugs prescribed by his doctor. But it did not occur to him to question their effects. How could he know they would enslave him?

Of 420 people queried about their drug habits, 43 percent said they or someone in their family or a close friend were addicted to drugs or alcohol.

In 1978 alone doctors prescribed Darvon 31 million times. Nearly 275 million prescriptions for tranquilizers are filled every year. Sixty million of these are for Valium.[4] A report from the Health and Science Research Committee of the United States alerted the American people, "If you require a daily dose of Valium to get through each day, you are hooked and you should seek help. No one is immune from the nightmare of dependence and addiction to these drugs. It affects doctors, clergy, teachers and laborers, business executives and housewives."[5]

Jeanne, a witty, attractive grandmother in her late sixties, has suffered from high blood pressure for thirty years. For twenty-five years she had taken a diuretic and high-blood-pressure medication. Recently she had repeated headaches and dizziness. Her doctor said her blood pressure was elevated. He gave her another prescription to add to her previous medication. Jeanne took the three prescription drugs for one month. When she complained to her doctor that she was tense and irritable, he added a drug that was new on the market, making a total of four pills. The day she picked up her medicine from the pharmacy she left on a trip.

A few days after arriving at her son and daughter-in-law's home, she became upset for no apparent reason. Every morning for five days the same thing happened. By midafternoon Jeanne would cry and be unable to control her emotions or disturbing thought patterns. She was afraid of losing her mind.

Her daughter-in-law, Ann, who is a registered nurse, asked what drugs she was taking. Ann made a list and looked them up in the *Physician's Desk Reference*. She found the side effects from these drugs were the same symptoms Jeanne was having. That afternoon, Ann took her to a doctor who took Jeanne off two of the medications. Within two days her hysteria disappeared and Jeanne was herself again. She wrote the names of the drugs in her notebook to make sure no one would prescribe them for her again.

In 1960 eighteen prescriptions were filled every second in

the U.S. The staggering cost of these pink, violet, yellow, white, and green tablets, capsules, lozenges, and ampules amounted to 3 billion dollars a year. In 1981 the figure had increased to 10 billion dollars.[6]

Mary is a young, vivacious registered nurse, married to a hard-working businessman who is admired and respected by his friends and acquaintances. They live in Indianapolis with their four-year-old son and five-year-old daughter. They attend church regularly and have many Christian friends.

During the early years of their marriage, Mary spent eighteen months in bed recovering from tuberculosis. Five years later migraine headaches attacked her. Dr. Ray, her internist, prescribed Caffergot for the headaches. She became tense and experienced deep anxiety. Librium, a tranquilizer was added. Depression set in, and Elavil, a mood elevator, was ordered. Her feet and hands swelled so a diuretic was prescribed. Her back began to ache, and Darvon was prescribed. The last straw was the onset of rheumatoid arthritis. The remedy for this was three aspirin every three hours. There was a pill for every ill. Her body became a walking laboratory. One day her mother told her, "Your personality has changed. I don't know you anymore."

How did this all happen? Mary didn't question her doctor because she was a nurse and had been taught not to question doctors. She thought all of the answers to her health problems lay in the field of medicine. Round and round she rode on her merry-go-round of prescription drugs.

Desperately she prayed for help. God spoke through His Word. "Don't get your stimulus from wine (for there is always the danger of excessive drinking), but let the Spirit stimulate your souls" (Ephesians 5:18 PHILLIPS). She was shocked as the thought struck: *I am drunk with prescription drugs. How can I be filled with the Spirit?*

As she searched God's Word for answers she also read 1 Corinthians 6:19–20 PHILLIPS: "Have you forgotten that your body is the temple of the Holy Spirit, who lives in you, and is God's gift to you, and that you are not the owner of your own body? You have been bought, and at what a price! Therefore bring glory to God in your body."

It was then that the idea hit her: *Beware of prescription drugs. They may be endangering your health.* The clarity of her thinking astonished her. She ran to her medicine cabinet, filled a paper bag with the drugs, and dumped them in the garbage can.

The next seven days were a nightmare of misery and suffering as her body slowly withdrew from its dependency on the drugs. But victory finally came.

Then she began to search for ways to improve her health. The program that appealed to her was something she would have to do herself—with God's help. Through the encouragement of several Christian friends, she developed a do-it-yourself program. The foundation of this program was prayer and studying God's Word. Through this effort she learned to relax in the Lord.

A nutritionist suggested a diet change. The new diet included many fresh vegetables and fruits, whole-grain breads and cereals, dairy products, nuts and seeds, high-quality proteins, and fewer fats. The books she read warned of the hazards of salt, sugar, and caffeine in excess, so these foods were eliminated from her diet.

Through a friend's urging she started a daily exercise program. A doctor friend suggested drinking water on a daily basis and taking vitamin and mineral supplements.

As she worked on these changes she started applying the promises she read in God's Word. Gradually her health improved. She didn't need any chemical crutches. I can identify strongly with this story, because I am Mary.[7]

If you are caught on a merry-go-round of pills, God can give you victory. Although healing comes from Him, the desire to take the initiative in assuming the responsibility for your own health is the first step.

All physicians are required to take the Hippocratic Oath, part of which reads: "I will neither give a deadly drug to anybody, if asked for it, nor will I make a suggestion to this effect." With this oath in my mind, a patient should feel free to ask specific questions about the drugs that are being prescribed. If it is necessary for you to take prescription drugs, ask your physician to list the benefits and side effects. Some drugs produce the same side effects as the indications. Ask if the drug is to cure the condition or only alleviate discomfort. Ask how long it will be before the drug shows the expected results. Evaluate the facts yourself: If the benefits of a drug outweigh the risks, you are safer.

You have a right to know precisely what goes into your body; it is, after all, the temple of the Holy Spirit.

Ask yourself these questions.

Are you taking any drugs, either prescription or over-the-counter? If not, what were the last drugs you took? List them.

1. _____

2. _____

3. _____

4. _____

How long? _____

Do you know what the drugs are given for?

1. _____

2. _____

3. _____

If two or more drugs are being taken, have you asked your doctor if they are compatible with each other? _____. Were they prescribed by the same doctor? _____. Do these drugs have a cumulative effect in your body? _____.

What are the side effects of the drugs you are taking?

1. _____

2. _____

3. _____

Are the side effects worse than the problem? _____.

Current research indicates certain drugs can react adversely with food and beverages. For example:

1. Calcium in milk and other dairy products impairs the absorption of tetracycline.[8]
2. Iron Supplements with fruit juice enhances absorption of iron.
3. Soda pop may cause excess acidity and dissolve drugs in the stomach instead of in the intestines.
4. Licorice can aggravate high blood pressure.
5. MAO Inhibitor drugs used for depression and high blood pressure can react with tyramine in aged cheese, chianti wine, and chicken livers causing high blood pressure, headaches, and brain hemorrhages. Other foods suspected of reacting with these drugs are salami, pepperoni, yogurt, bananas, avocados, sour cream, cola beverages, coffee, chocolate, and raisins.
6. Alcohol combined with antibiotics, anticoagulants, diabetic drugs, antihistamines, high-blood-pressure drugs (MAO Inhibiters), and sedatives can cause extreme drowsiness and be hazardous.
7. Colchicine, a drug prescribed for gout, and mineral oil, an ingredient in some over-the-counter laxatives, can cause faulty nutrient absorption.
8. The drug INH can cause a B6 deficiency.
9. Diuretics can lead to serious potassium depletion.
10. Chronic use of antacids can cause phosphate depletion, which produces muscle weakness and vitamin-D deficiency.
11. The pill (oral contraceptives) can lower folic acid and B12 levels in the blood.[9]

Are you taking any of the above mentioned drugs? _____.
Name them:

1. _____

2. _____

3. _____

What foods should you eliminate or increase in your diet while taking these drugs?

_____

_____

_____

4   PERSONAL LIFESTYLE CHECKUP

Because I want this book to reach you personally, let us pretend you have come to me for a nutritional consultation. On the telephone before you come, I will ask you to fill out and return the health-diet questionnaire that will be forwarded to you. We will go over the questions as they appear on the form. Use the space between them for your personal lifestyle checkup. I am teaching you to be your own nutritional advisor so you can assume responsibility for your own health. (Get a pencil and extra paper.)

HEALTH QUESTIONNAIRE

1. Statement of present health in your own words:

_____

_____

_____

2. Past surgery, accidents, injuries, or medical illness:

_____

_____

_____

3. List medications, vitamins, and minerals you take regularly:

_____

_____

_____

4. Habits (check and specify amount)

☐ Alcohol _____

☐ Tobacco _____

☐ Coffee _____

Please check and give dates if you have or ever had:

☐ _____ Rheumatic Fever
☐ _____ Swollen or Painful Joints
☐ _____ Frequent or Severe Headaches
☐ _____ Dizziness or Fainting Spells
☐ _____ Cramps in Legs
☐ _____ Gall-bladder Trouble
☐ _____ Piles or Rectal Disease
☐ _____ Venereal Disease
☐ _____ Paralysis (Inc. Polio)
☐ _____ Frequent or Painful Urination
☐ _____ Excessive Drinking Habit
☐ _____ Ear, Nose, or Throat Trouble
☐ _____ Chronic or Frequent Colds

☐ _____ Severe Tooth or Gum Trouble
☐ _____ Palpitation or Pounding Heart
☐ _____ High or Low Blood Pressure
☐ _____ Pain or Pressure in Chest
☐ _____ Shortness of Breath
☐ _____ Loss of Memory or Amnesia
☐ _____ Chronic Cough
☐ _____ Frequent Indigestion
☐ _____ Gall Stones
☐ _____ Back Problems
☐ _____ Sugar or Albumin in Urine
☐ _____ Frequent Trouble Sleeping
☐ _____ Recent Weight Change
☐ _____ Depression or Excessive Worry

☐ _____ Drug or Narcotic Habit	☐ _____ Liver or Intestinal Trouble
☐ _____ Sinusitis	☐ _____ Heart Trouble
☐ _____ Hay Fever	☐ _____ Neuritis
☐ _____ Jaundice	☐ _____ Epilepsy or Fits
☐ _____ Goiter	☐ _____ Kidney Stone
☐ _____ Tuberculosis	☐ _____ Blood in Urine
☐ _____ Asthma	☐ _____ Nervous Trouble
☐ _____ Stomach Trouble	

Now read the answers you wrote. Think about each one, then review the previous chapters. Do you see any correlation between your problems and some of the statistics in the previous chapters? Check out the risk factors. Are you in a high-risk category? Are you getting some clues to possible causes of your health problems? List any thoughts or ideas you come up with.

_____

_____

_____

_____

_____

The danger of writing this type of book is that I will put myself out of business when you learn to be your own nutritionist. Yet the only way any of us can be successful is to multiply ourselves. To have you take your nutrition seriously is my ultimate goal and purpose for writing this book.

My aim is not to tell you what to do with any illnesses you have; that is your physician's job. My job is to teach you how to prevent or avoid health problems you don't yet have. Prevention techniques can often positively affect an illness you already have.

The last part of your questionnaire will ask you to give

dietary information. *This is very important.* Many prospective patients refuse, and I refuse to counsel them. If you will not take the time to think about what you eat and list it on paper, you will not be disciplined enough to follow a nutrition program. Many prospective patients filled it in, and when they gave it to me and said, "I am so ashamed for you to see what I eat," I knew I could work with these people. They had already learned how dreadful their diet was and knew they needed to make changes.

I. DIET CHECKUP

List your *typical daily* diet for *each meal* on page 31. List all the food you eat for a period of one week. Include all between meal snacks. *Be specific* and use a separate sheet of paper if necessary.

Study your seven-day diet sheet carefully. Ask yourself:

1. How many meals do I eat a day? _____.

2. If I skip any, which ones? _____.

3. How do I feel when I skip a meal? _____.

4. If I skip breakfast, does it matter? _____. (Would you try to drive your car to work on an empty fuel tank?)

There is a saying, "Eat a breakfast fit for a king, lunch fit for a prince, and supper fit for a pauper." How do my meals stack up against this saying?

List meal fit for a king _____.

For a prince _____.

For a pauper _____.

Statistics show that in 50 percent of American families one or more persons skip breakfast entirely. In 40 percent of the families, the children are responsible for their own breakfasts.

	Breakfast	Dinner	Supper	Snacks
MONDAY	_____	_____	_____	_____
TUESDAY	_____	_____	_____	_____
WEDNESDAY	_____	_____	_____	_____
THURSDAY	_____	_____	_____	_____
FRIDAY	_____	_____	_____	_____
SATURDAY	_____	_____	_____	_____
SUNDAY	_____	_____	_____	_____

1. Are your snacks nourishing? _____. List them:

_____

_____

2. Is the food high quality? _____. List types:

_____

_____

_____

3. List the low-quality foods:

_____

_____

_____

4. Is the quantity too much or too little? _____.

5. Is your diet high or low in calories? _____.

6. Is your diet high in fat? _____.

7. Do you eat much sugar? Check and see. In what?

_____

_____

_____

8. Do you get any fiber each day? _____. (Whole grains, beans, nuts, seeds, vegetables, fruits, raw foods.)

9. Could your diet be stressing your body? How?

_____

_____

_____

_____

10. Where and how can you improve your diet?

_____

_____

_____

_____

_____

II. WATER CONSUMPTION CHECKUP

Write down how many glasses of water you drink each day.

Glasses of water: _____.

Daily Water-Consumption Formula:
Take one-half of your body weight; multiply by 80 percent. This gives you the total ounces of water you need each day.[1]

How much should you drink? _____.

III. EXERCISE CHECKUP

Do you exercise? _____. What kind? _____

How often (number of days per week)? _____. How long each time (minutes)? _____

IV. REST AND RELAXATION CHECKUP

How many hours of sleep do you get each night? _____.

Are you rested when you get up? _____.

How much time do you spend relaxing each day? _____.

What do you do to relax? _____

Keep this information you have compiled for reference as you read the remaining chapters.

Hippocrates, the Father of Medicine, said, "A wise man should consider that health is the greatest of human blessings and learn how by his own thought to derive benefit from his illness."[2]

A friend, who is a physician, heard me speak and tell about my history of poor health in my younger years. Afterward he remarked, "You have the secret to good health and long life." I asked, "What do you mean?" He replied, "If everyone could get a disease early in life that doesn't kill them, but brings with it a solution that causes them to form good habits and build self-discipline, the chances are that they will live a long life."

My husband is a good example. When he was thirteen he was run over by a car and suffered a ruptured spleen, which had to be surgically removed. He was told to take good care of himself because his immune system would never be as strong as before. When he was nineteen years old and a freshman in college, he had a hemorrhaging duodenal ulcer that nearly ended his life. He was cured medically and told to never smoke or drink alcohol and to watch his diet carefully. Further advice was to get plenty of rest and learn to deal with stress. We have had thirty blessed years of marriage together and are looking forward to the next thirty. Alfred Lord Tennyson said, "Oh, yet we trust that somehow good will be the final goal of ill."[3]

5   LET'S SET SOME GOALS

Before you read this chapter, I want to be the first to tell you, "You *can* do it!" Now, repeat aloud after me: "I can do it. I can do it. I can do all things through Him [Christ] who strengthens me" (Philippians 4:13).

Do what? Substitute health-giving habits for detrimental habits. Zig Ziglar says, "When you're going after Moby Dick, put tartar sauce in your boat."[1] He also says, "If you had a half-million dollar race horse, would you keep him up drinking coffee, alcohol, and smoking all night like you do yourself? . . . Would you feed your dog junk food?"[2]

Health doesn't just happen. It requires planning. And exercise, nutritious food, and good sleep are all a part of the plan. As we try to establish new health goals for ourselves, we should remember the words of Jonathan Swift: "The best doctors in the world are Dr. Diet, Dr. Quiet, and Dr. Merryman."[3] Dr. Exercise is important as well.

To help you understand these goals, let us review a case history from my office files. The patient, in this case, is "extra special" because he is a relative of mine. I'll call him Lee.

One day the phone rang. It was Lee's wife calling from Indiana. In a tearful voice she said, "Lee made it through the surgery fine, but the prognosis is poor. He has squamous-cell carcinoma of the lung, and it is entangling the aorta artery. They could remove only about half of it." Her voice broke and she said, "What are we going to do? The doctor said he has from six months to a year to live."

I knew how serious this was. It had been only five years since another family member had died of cancer (carcinoma of the colon). Now we were faced with another relative going through this devastating illness.

I responded, "Let's pray about it; we'll call you back later."

My husband, son, daughter, and I began to ask the Lord

what we could do to help Lee and his wife. We asked for wisdom for Lee in the decisions he would have to make about his treatment. We called friends for additional prayer support. One answer seemed to be to do a nutritional profile and diet survey to develop a nutritional program for Lee. To do this, we flew to Indiana to see Lee and his wife.

On our flight from Arizona, my husband and I were reviewing Lee's lifestyle to see what changes had to be made. As we discussed his diet and habits, we recognized the pattern. He loved fatty foods of all kinds. Meat was a big part of his diet— and the fatter, the better. He loved pork and shellfish too. Breakfast was always bacon, eggs, toast, and lots of coffee. He would eat vegetables but didn't go out of his way to get them. He seldom ate fruit. He never drank water. One thing he didn't eat was sweets; he didn't care for desserts. Lee had been a heavy smoker for over fifty years and enjoyed his cocktails daily.

Everyone loved Lee because of his winsome personality. He would always put himself out to help people. In business he was a hard driver and extremely productive and successful. When a crisis came, he would become tense and upset. He often worried that things would turn out wrong, and he fought a negative mental attitude his whole life. He got little exercise or relaxation to help his body function better. As Lee grew older he began to tire more easily and often went to bed as soon as dinner was over.

My concern was whether he would be willing to follow the program I would give him. Some of my suggestions I had learned when I accompanied my husband to Europe. I visited doctors in Germany and interviewed them about the nutrition programs they used with their cancer patients, and they shared the specifics of such treatments and the rate of success. I had used their suggestions before with people who had cancer.

After sharing hugs and tears with Lee and his wife, we sat down and discussed the problem they were facing. Lee said, "One of my doctors suggested radiation therapy, but I haven't decided yet. I talked with another doctor, an old friend, and he said, 'Go fishing for a month and think about it before you decide.' They say there isn't anything else they can do for me that might help."

Then I said, "Lee, after all of us had spent time in prayer and asked for prayer support from our church and friends, we came to one conclusion. Everything that can be done to build up your body should be started before radiation or anything else."

Then I showed him and his wife the program I had developed. We set some goals—his *Dr. Diet Goals:*

1. Eat whole-grain breads and cereals.
2. Eat fresh vegetables, both raw and cooked in large quantities every day. Drink carrot juice often.
3. Use fruit for snacks.
4. Combine beans and rice, or corn and beans, or eat lentils, split peas, or soybean products to replace some of the meat.
5. Use fish, chicken, and turkey in small quantities to replace red meat. Eat very little red meat.
6. Use only low-fat dairy products and only in small amounts.
7. Cut out fat, coffee, smoking, and alcohol.
8. Each day use bran for extra fiber.
9. Use very little table salt.
10. Drink eight glasses of water each day.
11. Continue the habit of not eating sweets.

For his *Dr. Exercise goals,* I suggested the following:

Walk slowly each day in the fresh air and build up to a program of two miles in thirty minutes.

To detoxify the body, take an enema made from four cups of weak coffee each day. Retain the solution for at least fifteen minutes each time.

This prompted a reaction. Lee said, "Why can't I just drink and enjoy the coffee?" I explained, "When you drink it, the effect is different. We want to use it to stimulate the portal vein of your liver to help remove toxic waste from your body."

Next, I explained that he would have to take vitamins,

minerals, and enzymes. Some of the supplements would have to be added after I returned to Phoenix and ran tests. That day he started his program of proteolytic enzymes, emulsified vitamin A, and vitamin C.

Lee said, "My goal is to get well, and I will do anything to feel better." His wife vowed: "I will do whatever it takes to help him."

After he had been on the nutrition program a short time, he started regaining some of the weight he had lost. He recovered from his surgery and looked healthier. His strength gradually increased.

He started to worry about whether he was really getting better and wondered if he would ever get well. His negative thoughts overwhelmed him, and he could only envision himself as a sick person. I called him from Arizona to remind him that his mind was a powerful factor in healing his body. I suggested he practice envisioning himself well and the cancer cells being destroyed. I also suggested he read some funny stories, be around happy, fun-filled people, and learn to laugh. In other words, I was encouraging him to spend more time with *Dr. Merryman*.

At the end of one month, he made the decision to go ahead with the radiation treatments. He finished a set of twenty-five treatments and had resultant burning of the esophagus, at which time we ran more tests and added more vitamins and minerals.

It has been seven months since his surgery. Lee has been fishing in Florida and recently drove two thousand miles to visit us in Arizona. We don't know the outcome of his illness, but at seventy-nine years of age, he is able to be up and around each day. There is quality to his life.

Dr. Quiet has the answer for the days he is very tired. He recuperates well with a nap. I told him to rest more and spend quiet times alone with the Lord.

Recently when Lee was X-rayed, his doctor reported the tumor had decreased so much that it was almost nonexistent. Since the bone scan was also negative, we are all rejoicing and continuing to pray for God's direction in his life, even though we don't know how much longer he has. Only God knows, but God has chosen, at least for now, to renew his health.

Take paper and pencil and let us work out some goals for you. Choose from the lists below where you want to start.

DR. DIET SUGGESTS:

1. Whole-grain breads and cereals.
2. Fresh vegetables—raw and cooked two or three times daily.
3. Vegetable juices (if available).
4. Fish, chicken, turkey, veal; only small amounts of beef and lamb.
5. Lentils, split peas, soybeans, beans and rice, and beans and corn instead of flesh protein at some meals.
6. Eggs limited to four a week.
7. Low-fat dairy products.
8. Fruit—fresh for snacks and dessert.
9. Less salt, sugar, caffeine, fats.

DR. MERRYMAN SUGGESTS:

1. Read the comics and humorous books.
2. Look for humor in life.
3. Laugh at yourself. (Don't take yourself so seriously.)
4. Smile—it's infectious.
5. Be with humorous people.
6. Watch funny movies and television shows.
7. Be positive in your mental attitude.
8. Say, "I can do it." ("I can do all things through Christ.")

DR. QUIET SUGGESTS:

1. Stop and smell the flowers.
2. Listen to others quietly.
3. Establish a daily quiet time for prayer and Bible reading.
4. Listen to relaxing music.
5. Walk in the woods (real or imaginary).
6. Listen to the birds.
7. Sit by the sea (real or imaginary).
8. Take a vacation and do something relaxing.
9. Lie down and take a nap.

DR. EXERCISE SUGGESTS:

Start slowly and build up your endurance.
Pick your exercise:

1. Walking (goal—two miles in 30 minutes).
2. Running or jogging—consult with your physician.
3. Rebounding on trampoline.
4. Bicycling.
5. Jumping rope.
6. Aerobics dance class.
7. Sports—and not as a spectator!
8. To develop and strengthen muscles, do specific exercises or weight lifting.

Dr. Diet's suggestions are good for about 90 percent of the population. Due to metabolism differences 10–20 percent may need more dietary fats than others. You may also find grains and fruits don't give you the energy you need. You may need to add more protein foods. See chapter 7 on how to find out which are best.

List the choices you have made for yourself in the Do-It-Yourself Nutrition Program.

DR. DIET'S GOAL

_____

_____

_____

DR. MERRYMAN'S GOAL

_____

_____

_____

DR. QUIET'S GOAL

_____

_____

_____

DR. EXERCISE'S GOAL

_____

_____

_____

Beware! Do not follow the directions of these doctors:

Dr. Junk Food
Dr. Grump or Dr. Grouch
Dr. Busybody
Dr. Sit Around

6 ARE YOU IN TUNE WITH YOUR BODY?

Do you know anything about your body's anatomy and physiology? When we need to make changes in our lives, it helps to know why. Let us examine the make-up of the human body and lay a foundation for later use.

Psalm 139:14 says, "I will give thanks to Thee, for I am fearfully and wonderfully made" (NASB). God has made each of us biologically individual, and yet we all have similarities.

Think about your body as we begin this discussion. The human body is a highly organized, single structure made up of billions of smaller structures called cells, tissues, membranes, glands, and systems.[1]

First, let us try to picture the systems of the body.

Q. What enables us to sit up, lie down, and move around?
A. The skeletal system, made up of bones, cartilage, and muscles, is responsible for support and movement.

Q. Why can we hear, see, smell, feel, and taste?
A. Because of the nervous system, which is made up of cells, sense organs, and the endocrine system. It gives us communication, control, and integration of the functioning parts of the body.

Q. What keeps the blood flowing and healthy?
A. The cardiovascular system, blood, and lymphatic systems are the body's transport system.

Q. What is responsible for building energy and waste removal?
A. The respiratory system, digestive system, and urinary system are responsible for the body's energy supply and waste excretion.

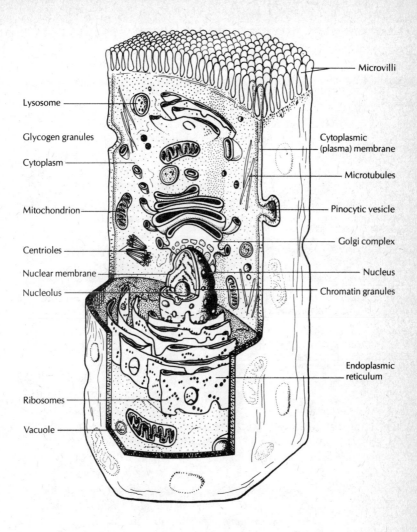

Lysosome

Glycogen granules

Cytoplasm

Mitochondrion

Centrioles

Nuclear membrane

Nucleolus

Ribosomes

Vacuole

Microvilli

Cytoplasmic (plasma) membrane

Microtubules

Pinocytic vesicle

Golgi complex

Nucleus

Chromatin granules

Endoplasmic reticulum

Fig 6.1. An artist's interpretation of cell structure as seen under an electron microscope. Note the many mitochondria, popularly known as the "power plants of the cell." Note, too, the innumerable dots bordering the endoplasmic reticulum. These are ribosomes, the cell's "protein factories." (Illustration by Louise Bauer)

Q. How can we reproduce ourselves?
A. The reproductive system, which is different for a male and female, allows this.

Q. What fights disease and heals our body?
A. The immune system is responsible for the body's defense against disease and stress.

Q. What distributes electrolytes and maintains fluid balance?
A. The fluid and electrolyte balance mechanism.

Q. What balances the acidity or alkalinity of the body fluids?
A. The acid-base balance mechanism. This balance is called PH and can be measured in the blood, urine, and saliva.

Look over these systems, and make sure they make sense. Think of your own bones, nerves, heart, and blood, and try to picture your lungs, stomach, colon, kidneys, bladder, and reproductive system. Envision your white blood cells uniting to destroy a foreign invader bacteria inside your body. Can you see the fluids (including water) that contain and move the various nutrients around? What causes acid indigestion after a big meal and what happens when you take an antacid or alkalizer?

Are you ready to move on to the fascinating world of cells? In 1925 E. B. Wilson said, "Long ago it became evident that the key to every biological problem must finally be sought in the cell; for every living organism is, or at some time has been a cell."[2]

The human body is a large structural unit made up of smaller parts. The smallest unit that can maintain life and reproduce is the cell.[3] Cells are made up of smaller parts arranged by the Creator in an orderly and precise manner. Organization is one of the most important characteristics of life and is clearly seen in cells. We need to protect our cells from ourselves.

Rudy, one of my nutritional counselees, is driven to my office by his wife. When he was a young boy his *optic nerve cells* were destroyed and he is blind. The rest of his body operates, but those nerve cells are dead.

Another young man, named Ed, is barely able to stand up

and walk by himself. His mumbled speech comes only after great effort to form each word. Some of his *brain cells were damaged* at birth, and he has cerebral palsy. He is intelligent and, with the help of a friend, writes stories from the depth of his emotions that move the reader to tears and challenge him to serve the Lord. Can you see how important our cells are to us? They are as important as the following equation: **Cellular Health = Tissue Health = Organ Health = System Health = Body Health.**[4]

The Psalmist writes, "For Thou didst form my inward parts; Thou didst weave me in my mother's womb" (Psalm 139:13 NASB). God is interested in the tiniest part of the smallest cell of our bodies, they are handmade by Him. "Thank you Lord, for my body. May I never take it for granted. As I look at these pictures of some types of cells, help me remember Your concern about every small detail of my life as well as Your concern for my body."

One of the systems of this "fearfully and wonderfully made body" that merits further discussion is the digestive system. But before we start, we should listen to Dr. Exercise and take a fifteen-minute break so we will be able to think better.

The National Digestive Disease Advisory Board says, "One hundred million Americans, almost half the population, occasionally suffer from some form of digestive illness. Today digestive diseases represent the leading cause for hospitalization and major surgery in this country, accounting for 15% of all hospitalizations, 25% of all operations other than tonsillectomies, $17 billion in medical bills. . . . About 20 million Americans suffer from ulcers—sores that develop along the lining of the gastrointestinal tract." They recommend, "At first symptoms or diagnosis of an ulcer, eliminate the foods that aggravate the symptoms, such as, caffeine, alcohol, acid-bearing foods—citrus fruits and their juices and aspirin."[5]

The report states, "Diverticulosis is created by the tiny pouches, called diverticula, that form along the wall of the large intestine becoming inflamed and causing pain. This condition is prevalent in America."[6]

Researchers cite evidence that the condition is virtually unknown in underdeveloped countries where the diet is high in roughage and unrefined grains.

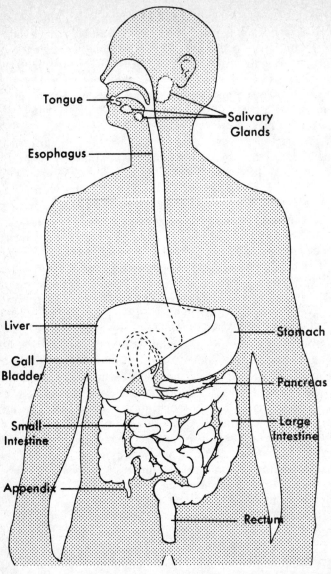

Fig 6.2. Location of digestive-system organs. (From John N. Moore and Harold S. Slusher, *Biology: A Search for Order in Complexity* [Grand Rapids: Zondervan, 1970], 286)

About 60 percent of the people I see in my office complain of digestive problems, and most of these problems are longstanding. The counselees said the digestive problem came first; then the arthritis, blood-sugar problem, heart problem, kidney problem, cancer, or some other condition followed. Could there be a correlation? A cause and effect?

By definition, digestion is the process by which food is converted into chemical and physical forms so that it can be absorbed and metabolized by the body.[7]

The organs of the digestive system start with the mouth and progress downward through the body. Next the salivary glands, teeth, pharynx, esophagus and stomach, then the small intestine, large intestine (colon), peritoneum, liver, gall bladder, and pancreas.

We eat six different kinds of substances, namely, carbohydrates, proteins, fats, vitamins, mineral salts, and water. Only the carbohydrates, proteins, and fats have to be chemically digested to be absorbed and metabolized. These three complex compounds unite with water and split into simple compounds; this process is called hydrolysis. Numerous enzymes present in the various digestive juices accelerate these chemical reactions and yet do not appear in the final product of the reaction. These enzymes are called organic catalysts.[8]

What about the three remaining substances—vitamins, mineral salts, and water—that come from digested foods? They are absorbed through the intestinal wall or mucosa into the blood and lymph transport system to be metabolized by the body.

I will single out the liver, the largest internal organ of the body and a part of the digestive system, because it is one of the most vital organs of the body. It has four main functions:

1. Liver cells take poisonous substances (drugs, alcohol, and other toxic compounds) that enter the blood through absorption from the small intestine and change them into nontoxic compounds. It serves as a detoxifier.

2. Liver cells secrete about a pint of bile a day. These bile salts aid in absorption of fats.

3. Liver cells help metabolize proteins, fats, and carbohydrates.

4. Liver cells store several substances: iron, and vitamins A, B_{12}, and D.[9]

All liver functions are important for health, But some of its metabolic processes are crucial for *survival itself*. Two examples follow.

We met Tom when we were living in Caracas, Venezuela, in 1956. Every time we were with him and his wife, he drank many cocktails, became intoxicated, and made a scene. We worried about his drinking habit. One day he became very ill, and the result of that illness was amputation of both his legs. But he kept on drinking. Later he had a heart attack. He continued to drink. A short time later, Tom's wife wrote and told us Tom had died from cirrhosis of the liver.

I met Jane when she was a patient in a clinic in Jamaica where I was doing cancer research. She had been operated on for pain in her upper right epigastrium. The diagnosis handed down after surgery was cancer of the liver caused by metastasis from a primary lesion in the stomach. She had come to Jamaica in hopes of finding something she could do to help herself. I kept in touch with her, but she lived only one more year.

Yes, the liver is a vital organ. You may have to read this chapter over several times before it sticks with you. Look over the information again and answer the following questions.

List the different systems of the body and what they are responsible for.

1. _____

_____

2. _____

_____

3. _____

_____

4. _____

_____

5. _____

_____

6. _____

_____

What are the two balance mechanisms listed and what are their functions?

1. _____

_____

2. _____

_____

What is a cell and its function?

_____

_____

Name some cells.

1. _____

_____

2. _____

_____

3. _____

_____

4. _____

_____

What is the equation showing the importance of cells?

_____

_____

What is digestion?

_____

Name some of the organs of the digestive system.

1. _____

2. _____

3. _____

What are the six kinds of substances present in food?

1. _____

2. _____

3. _____

4. _____

5. _____

6. _____

Name one of the largest and most important organs of the body.

_____

Why is it so important? Name four functions.

_____

1. _____

2. _____

3. _____

4. _____

7 LET'S GO TO THE MOON
(DON'T FORGET WATER, CARBOHYDRATES, FATS, AND PROTEINS)

In the field of nutrition today, there is much conflicting advice. Because many of the theories are complicated, people frequently tell me they are puzzled and don't know what to believe about the foods they should eat. But I believe God has made it simple. Man has made it difficult. So let us sort out the pieces of the nutrition puzzle so that we can restructure our thinking.

To piece together the fundamentals of nutrition, let us imagine we are going to the moon with Neil Armstrong. It is July 16, 1969, and we are prepared for take-off. Let us run down our check-list of essential items for supporting life during our trip. Our spaceship is properly pressurized and equipped to maintain a suitable temperature for the human body.

Since our bodies do not store oxygen, we must have an adequate supply on board, or we would die. After oxygen, what would be our most important priority? Did you guess food? Actually, it would be water. Without it, a normal healthy person can only live a few days. This is because our bodies are about two-thirds water: our blood is 90 percent water, and muscles contain 75–80 percent water.[1] Our intake of water must equal our output, or excretion, because the human body is a water-cooled machine.[2]

Water solutions carry the nutrients in food to the living cells and take the waste away. Life and health depend on a sufficient amount of water to replenish the daily losses from the body. So we must take an adequate water supply for our trip.

The next necessary item would be food, though for a short trip we could live without it. A strong man can live off his fuel reserve without eating for several weeks. I do not, however, advocate long fasts. Under careful supervision, I have seen many people improve their health by short periods of fasting. Even then, most experts agree that fasting with fruit and vegetable juices is the most beneficial. We do not live off the food we eat, but off the energy in the food we eat. Food is used to build fuel and provide additional water for our bodies. The food supply must contain adequate protein, fats, carbohydrates, vitamins, and minerals for our needs.

The next essential part of our trip to the moon would be an exercise program developed for limited space.

These, then, are the basic necessities. Now, let us dig deeper and learn more about the first two: water and food.

Typical normal values for each portal of water entry and exit (with wide variations)

Intake		Output	
Ingested liquids	1,500 ml	Kidneys (urine)	1,400 ml
Water in foods	700 ml	Lungs (water in expired air)	350 ml
Water formed by catabolism	200 ml	Skin	
		By diffusion	350 ml
		By sweat	100 ml
		Intestines (in feces)	200 ml
Totals	2,400 ml		2,400 ml

WATER

A fashionable young woman named Sarah came into my office one day. Her major complaint was a problem with her complexion; her face was quite broken out. She said, "I've been to several skin doctors and taken antibiotics for this problem. Nothing seems to help, and I'm frustrated. Could you help me through nutrition?" After reviewing her diet and asking a multitude of questions, I asked, "Sarah, how much water do you drink?" She said, "Hardly any; I don't like water." I told her it would take me a week to work up a full program for her, but I asked her to drink, in the meantime, a total of one and three-fourths quarts of water daily, only five ounces at a time, but frequently during the day. This is how much water a 130-pound woman should drink each day. I wanted to see what would happen after a week of this regimen. Since her nutritional program hadn't been worked up yet, this was the only change we made.

At the end of the week, she returned. When she walked through the door of my office, I noticed her radiant smile. She said, "Look at my skin, it cleared up shortly after I started drinking the water daily." I knew then that she would continue to be faithful with her water drinking and would probably follow the nutritional program I had designed.

I have observed many changes in people's lives just from drinking water: constipation problems have been helped; children who have been constantly plagued with sore throats and colds have gotten better; and chronic bladder problems have been improved.

But there is a problem. Research has proved that our God-given water supply has been disastrously polluted throughout the earth. Statistics show that the drinking water in many towns and cities in our country, even though it is chemically treated, still contains harmful bacteria and viruses.

In 1978 federal health officials reported thirty-two water-borne disease outbreaks affecting 11,435 Americans.[3] In 1982 three city wells had to be closed in the area where I live because of contamination by harmful bacteria.[4] Before the situation was discovered, many people became ill. Some of the diseases listed by researchers linked to drinking water are heart disease from soft water and cancer from chemicals known to be carcinogenic, which are either there by accident or added to purify it. The Environmental Protection Agency conducted a survey of eighty cities that revealed cancer-causing chemicals in water systems throughout the country.

What can we do? Should we stop drinking water until water treatment plants solve the problem? No, we need to take matters into our own hands. One answer is to purchase home distillation units (steam is best) and make our own pure water. Steam-purified water can also be purchased in bottles. Since this water is mineral free, those who drink it should take a low-dose trace-mineral tablet daily or add two or three teaspoons of sea water to each quart. There are also purifiers with carbon blocks and activated carbon granules that can be used to filter drinking water. Although these units remove chemicals, a problem arises from not changing the filters often enough, which allows bacteria to grow and contaminate the water. Another alternative is to buy bottled water that has been filtered through activated carbon granules, then ozonized to sterilize it. Spring water from a rural area, where few pollutants can reach it, is another good water source. If you are buying bottled water, call the company and ask for the results of recent bacterial tests and inquire how often these tests are run.

What action will you take to make sure you have a safe water supply?

_____

_____

Do you have a water softener? _____. The water from this type of unit should never be used for drinking. It is extremely high is sodium.

How much water should you drink each day? (See the formula in chapter 4: ½ body weight × .80 = _____ ounces or _____ quarts.)

Never drink large glasses of water at one time. You want to flush the kidneys, not flood them. Drink only four to five ounces of water every thirty to sixty minutes repeatedly during the day.

FOOD

The food that God designed for our bodies is made up of carbohydrates, fats, and proteins. First, *carbohydrates* are made up of three elements: carbon, hydrogen, and oxygen. Carbohydrates are starches and sugars, and the chief source of energy for all body functions. Carbohydrates come in two forms: *complex* and *simple*. Examples of complex carbohydrates are unrefined grains, beans, vegetables, and fruits. Ounce for ounce, they have the same calorie content as protein and less than half the calories in fat. They also provide dietary fiber and are the *only* foods not linked to any of the leading killer diseases.[5]

Simple carbohydrates are found in highly refined grains, sugars, and juices. Because they are high in calories and low in nutrients, they are often called "naked calorie" foods and are suspected of causing a wide variety of common health problems.[6]

For example, Dr John Yudkin, author of *Sweet and Dangerous,* claims that a diet high in sugar is the most important dietary cause of clogged arteries and heart disease. He mentions two separate research studies that showed evidence that a high-sugar diet caused a significant increase in the fat levels in blood. The greatest increase was in the triglycerides, which are the kinds of blood fat that can promote the development of atherosclerosis.[7]

Does sugar as well as fat and salt promote heart disease in our bodies?

In 1875 the average American consumed about 40 pounds of sugar a year. Today average consumption has risen to about 128 pounds per person annually. Studies have shown how immigrants, who rarely ate sweets in their native countries, developed diabetes after adopting a Westernized diet high in sugar.[8] Dentists often link sugar with tooth decay and advise patients to greatly restrict their consumption of sweets. Both diabetes and hypoglycemia show a direct relationship to the diet consumed, and a sugar-free diet is suggested for both of these conditions.

Obesity is another problem related to sugar. By eating sweets, you can easily overload on calories before you are full. A person can consume the total daily calorie quota in one bag of candy.

Edna, a middle-aged, retired secretary, is an example. She came to my office asking me to help her lose weight. As I reviewed her diet sheet, I noticed she listed only ice cream under snacks. She had written in the margin, "I eat ice cream every afternoon and before going to bed every night." I silently calculated the hidden calories she was adding each day. So I challenged her, "Edna, how would you feel about substituting a small piece of fruit or raw vegetables for your ice-cream snacks?" She replied, "Why, I couldn't live without my ice cream." Then I said, "If you are sincere about wanting to lose weight, at least give it a try." She reluctantly agreed. I asked her to call me and report each week on how she was doing.

One week later her joyous voice rang out through the phone: "I haven't had any ice cream for seven days, and I have lost three pounds. It hasn't been easy, but I will try it again next week." Each week she reported that she had lost more weight. When she came in one month later, she looked slimmer and had a bounce to her step. "I never realized how much ice cream I was carrying around; I've jumped over that hurdle at least." Now she was ready to make additional diet changes.

We substituted lower-calorie foods for her usual high-calorie foods. After two more months, she came in for a review. I could not believe my eyes. I exclaimed, "You are a beautiful lady. You could be a fashion model." She had lost a total of twenty-five pounds in three months and had experienced the feeling of success. Her whole appearance had changed. She said, "It sure has been fun to buy new clothes, but the best thing is the way I feel. I have the energy now to enjoy life." She added, "You know, I've been a widow over seven years, and last week I was asked out by an old friend. We went out to dinner." With a twinkle in her eye, she said, "After dinner he asked me if I would like dessert. I saw ice cream on the menu and said politely, 'No thanks, I really don't care for desserts.' I don't even like ice cream anymore."

Examine your own diet sheet and list the complex carbohydrates written there.

_____

_____

Now write the simple or refined carbohydrates listed on your diet sheet.

Do you think you need to cut down on simple carbohydrate consumption? _____.

Are you overweight? _____.

Do you have unstable energy levels? _____.

How do sweets affect you? _____

Fats and *lipids* are another basic component of food. They are the most concentrated sources of energy in our diet. Fats furnish more than twice as many calories per gram as carbohydrates and proteins. In addition to providing energy, they act as carriers for the fat-soluble vitamins A, D, E, and K.[9]

There are three types of fatty acids: saturated, monounsaturated, and polyunsaturated.

Saturated fatty acids are found in such foods as butter, cheese, chocolate, coconut oil, meat, lard, pork, cream, milk, and poultry. Animal fats contain a large amount of saturated fatty acids. The more saturated a fat is, the firmer it is at room temperature. These fats are accused of raising the blood cholesterol level. Cholesterol is present in foods such as eggs and organ meats, our bodies also manufacture it.

Unsaturated fatty acids are made up of *monounsaturated* fats found in avocados, almonds, cashews, olives, most margarines, peanuts, peanut butter, and cottonseed and olive oils.

Polyunsaturated fats are found in pecans, walnuts, corn oil, fish, most soft margarines, mayonnaise, salad dressing, and cottonseed, safflower, soybean, sesame, and sunflower oils.

The late Nathan Pritikin, who was director of the Longevity Center in Santa Monica, California, believed unsaturated fats lower cholesterol levels in the blood. He said, "However, they create havoc by raising triglyceride levels and creating metabolic suffocation by resultant sludge in the blood." Most animal and vegetable fats are triglycerides.[10]

Dr. William Castelli, director of the Framingham Heart Study, estimates that half the women and two-thirds of the men in the United States should eat less saturated fat and cholesterol.[11]

Dr. Samuel Epstein, professor at the School of Public Health, University of Illinois Medical Center, Chicago, states, "As far as dietary fat is concerned, there is no question that a very wide range of environmental carcinogens, particularly pesticides and industrial chemicals, are fat soluble and are likely to accumulate in the food chain. So the more animal and dairy product fat you eat, the greater will be your intake of these fat-soluble carcinogens. It is also known, that high-fat and high-calorie diets increase the incidence of cancers in animals fed known carcinogens, and that low-fat diets seem to protect against cancer."[12]

The Senate's Select Committee on Nutrition and Human Needs recommended in 1977 that Americans reduce their fat intake from 42 percent of total calories to 30 percent. The committee suggested that we reduce saturated fats from 16 percent to 10 percent of our diet and cut our cholesterol intake from 600 milligrams per day to 300.[13] Other research groups advise cutting all dietary fat to as low as 10 to 15 percent of total calories.

Why don't researchers always agree about how much fat to eliminate from our diets? I believe it is because God designed each of us biochemically different. It is my opinion that 80 to 90 percent of us need a low-fat diet of only 10 to 15 percent fats. The other 10 to 20 percent of the population seem to be able to handle a diet composed of 30 percent fat calories including saturated fats.

Review the current disease statistics in chapter 2 and think about modern diet trends. Is there any correlation in your mind between the two?

Look back over your diet and list the foods containing saturated fats.

_____

_____

Then list the foods in your diet that contain unsaturated fats.

_____

_____

Do you have high blood pressure, heart disease, or cancer? _____.

Does anyone in your family have these diseases? _____.

Are your cholesterol and triglyceride blood studies elevated? _____.

How do you feel when you eat extremely fatty foods? _____

_____

Do you need to cut down your fat intake?

Saturated _____.

Unsaturated _____.

How will you do this?

_____

_____

Protein is the next major category of food. Second to water, protein is the most plentiful substance in the body. It is the major source of building material for muscles, bones, blood, skin, hair, nails, and internal organs, including the heart and brain. The largest group of proteins are those that catalyze reactions, namely, enzymes. There are nearly two thousand of these. Many hormones are made from protein as well.

During digestion the large molecules of proteins are broken down into simpler units called amino acids. The body requires twenty-two amino acids to make human protein. All but nine of these amino acids can be produced by the body. The nine that cannot be produced are called *essential amino acids* and must be provided by food, for if just one is missing, even temporarily, protein synthesis will be altered.[14]

There are two types of proteins. *Complete proteins* contain all of the essential amino acids and are found mostly in meats and dairy products. Some fish have little methionine, and milk protein is short on arginine. These two partially complete proteins are usually eaten with foods containing the missing amino acids. But remember, many of the complete-protein foods are high in *fat*.

Incomplete proteins are lacking or low in one of the essential amino acids, hence the term, "incomplete." The sources for these are mostly vegetables, fruits, and grains. Generally, these foods are low in fat.

Complete proteins can be obtained by combining different sources of incomplete protein, but it takes planning. Here is a guide. (By "legumes" we mean soybeans, peanuts, blackeyed peas, kidney beans, chickpeas, navy beans, pinto, and lima beans.)

Rice with either: Wheat
                                Legumes
                                Sesame seeds

Wheat with either: Legumes
                                Soybeans and peanuts
                                Soybeans and sesame seeds
                                Rice and soybeans

Legumes with either:	Corn
	Rice
	Wheat
	Sesame seeds
	Barley
	Oats
Fish with either:	Grains
	Legumes
Milk with:	Grains

Amino acids are the building blocks of protein. They are nitrogen-containing chemicals essential to life itself. The nine essential amino acids are methionine, threonine, *tryptophan,* isoleucine, leucine, *lysine,* histidine, valine, and phenylalanine. I have italicized the ones I will refer to in a later chapter. These are the celebrities focused on in current nutrition research as being directly connected with some current health disturbances.

Write down these two amino acids and familiarize yourself with them for later discussion.

1. _____

2. _____

Do you wonder what percentage of your diet should be protein? Because of its starring role in the drama called "The Human Body," protein has claimed center stage for many years. We often overreact by consuming twice as much protein as our bodies need, and as a result, excess protein can cause kidney damage, increase body fat, and cause the body to lose precious minerals such as calcium, iron, zinc, phosphorus, and magnesium.

The Food and Nutrition Board of the National Academy of Science has established *Recommended Daily Allowances* for protein intake, which are overestimated by 45 percent to allow for a margin of safety. Some researchers feel that four out of five of us could operate well on a third less than the RDA requirement.

Urea is the chief nitrogenous constituent of urine and final product of protein metabolism in the body. Its excess is one of the causes of uremia. The amount of urea excreted varies directly with the amount of protein in the diet.[15]

For four years I have run urea experiments from the urine of my nutritional clients. The results have indicated the presence of excess urea or protein waste in nearly 90 percent of all the people tested. By carefully studying their dietary protein consumption and cutting down on the amount of animal protein consumed each day, I have seen remarkable changes occur in the well-being of these people.

My conclusion is that most of us eat *too much* animal protein. Three to four ounces of animal protein plus vegetable proteins, dairy products, grains, beans, and eggs should provide adequate protein for the average person each day, although pregnant women, nursing mothers, and growing children need more than the average adult.

Analyze the protein foods in your diet for the coming week. Leave a space after each food so the gram amounts can be filled in.

Day 1 _____

_____

Day 2 _____

_____

Day 3 _____

_____

Day 4 _____

Day 5 _____

_____

Day 6 _____

_____

Day 7 _____

_____

Use the following chart to see how many grams of protein are in the foods you listed. Then add up your daily total: _____

PROTEIN IN "PROTEIN" FOODS[16]

Food	Serving size	Grams protein
Bacon	2 medium slices	3.8
Beef, chuck roast	3 ounces cooked	24.0
Beef, lean ground	¼ pound raw	23.4
Bologna	3 slices (3 ounces)	10.2
Cheese, American	1-ounce slice	6.6
Cheese, cheddar	1 ounce	7.1
Cheese, cottage	½ cup	15.0
Chicken, fryer	1 drumstick	12.2
Eggs	2 medium	11.4
Fish sticks	3 sticks (3 ounces)	14.1
Flounder	3 ounces	25.5
Frankfurter	1 (2 ounces)	7.1
Ham, boiled	3 slices (3 ounces)	16.2
Kidney, beef	½ cup cooked	23.1
Lamb, rib chop	3 ounces	17.9
Liver, chicken	1 liver	6.6
Mackerel	3 ounces	18.6

BLUEPRINT FOR HEALTH

Food	Serving size	Grams protein
Milk, skim	1 cup	8.8
Peanut butter	2 tablespoons	8.0
Pizza, cheese	¼ 14-inch pie	15.6
Pork, loin	3 ounces	20.8
Pork sausage	2 links (2 ounces)	5.4
Scallops	3 ounces fried	16.0
Shrimp	3 ounces fried	11.6
Tuna, canned	3 ounces drained	24.4
Turkey	3 ounces	26.8
Veal, stew meat	3 ounces	23.7
Yogurt	1 cup	8.3

PROTEIN IN OTHER FOODS[17]

Food	Serving size	Grams protein
Banana	1 medium	1.3
Barley	¼ cup raw	4.1
Bean curd (tofu)	1 piece	9.4
Beans, kidney	½ cup cooked	7.2
Beans, lima	½ cup cooked	6.5
Beans, navy	½ cup cooked	7.4
Bean sprouts (Mung)	½ cup	2.0
Bran flakes (40%)	1 cup	3.6
Bread, rye	1 slice	2.3
Bread, white	1 slice	2.4
Bread, whole wheat	1 slice	2.6
Broccoli	½ cup	2.4
Bulgur	1 cup cooked	8.4
Corn	½ cup kernels	2.7
Farina	1 cup cooked in water	3.2
Lentils	½ cup cooked	7.8
Macaroni	1 cup cooked	6.5
Muffin, corn	1 medium	2.8
Noodles, egg	1 cup cooked	6.5
Oatmeal	1 cup cooked in water	4.8
Pancakes	3 4-inch cakes	5.7

Food	Serving size	Grams protein
Peas, green	½ cup cooked	4.3
Potato	7 ounces baked	4.0
Rice, brown	1 cup cooked	4.9
Rice, white	1 cup cooked	4.1
Sesame seeds	1 tablespoon	1.5
Soup, bean with pork	1 cup with water	8.0
Soup, chicken noodle	1 cup with water	3.4
Soup, cream of mushroom	1 cup with milk	6.9
Soup, tomato	1 cup with milk	6.5
Soup, vegetable	1 cup with water	2.2
Soybeans	½ cup cooked	9.9
Spaghetti	1 cup cooked al dente	6.5
Squash, acorn	1 cup baked	3.9
Sweet potato	5 ounces baked	2.4
Walnuts	10 large	7.3
Wheat flakes	1 cup	3.1
Wheat, shredded	2 biscuits	5.0

Using the "Daily Recommended Dietary Allowance (RDA) for Protein" chart on the next page, calculate how many grams of protein the National Academy of Sciences says you need daily. Remember, you could probably cut it down by one-third. Write your answer here. _____.

Example: Find your age bracket, write down how much you weigh, multiply that by the number opposite your age bracket. A twenty-year-old adult who weighs 120 pounds would need 43.2 grams of protein daily.

    120 pounds
  × .36
    43.2 grams of protein daily

Now cutting this down to one-third, we get 28.8 grams. Are you eating more or less protein than you came up with? _____.

Work out the changes you will make.

DAILY RECOMMENDED DIETARY
ALLOWANCE (RDA) FOR PROTEIN[18]

Ages (in years)	Grams protein (per pound ideal body weight)
Infants	
0–0.5	1.00
0.5–1	0.90
Children	
1–3	0.81
4–6	0.68
7–10	0.55
11–14	0.45
15–18	0.39
Adults	
19 and over	0.36
Pregnant women	0.62
Nursing women	0.53

Note: Here are some sample calculations to determine a day's protein needs:

For a five-year-old child who weighs 50 pounds: $0.68 \times 50 = 34$ grams.

For a 160-pound man: $0.36 \times 160 = 57.6$ grams.

For a 110-pound twelve-year old: $0.45 \times 110 = 49.5$ grams.

For a 125-pound pregnant woman: $0.62 \times 125 = 77.5$ grams.

According to the Food and Nutrition Board of the National Academy of Sciences, the amounts of protein determined in this fashion should be adequate to meet the needs of virtually all healthy people.

8

DISCOVERING A WONDERFUL WORLD (VITAMINS, MINERALS, ENZYMES, AND FIBER)

John Goodwin, vice-president of the Agriculture Department at the University of Arkansas, fights what he calls agricultural illiteracy. He says, "Since the end of World War II the nation's relationship to farming has changed. Then about 85% of the people were only one generation removed from the land. Today the figure has dropped to 15%. . . . The 85% who are far removed from the land include people convinced milk comes from plastic cartons or containers. They do not realize that somebody milked a cow to get it."[1]

In this world of TV dinners, canned biscuits, slice-and-bake cookies, and instant everything, could we have fallen into the 85 percent who are agriculturally illiterate?

Can you come up with at least one source for each of the following?

Vitamins _____

Minerals _____

Enzymes _____

Fiber _____

When we think of vitamins, minerals, enzymes, and fiber we should picture gardens of vegetables and fruits; fields of grain, legumes, and nuts; animals, fish, and fowl in their natural habitat. If we picture shelves in a drug store, health-food store, or supermarket neatly displaying an array of bottles labeled vitamin supplement, mineral supplement, digestive enzymes, and dietary-fiber supplement, we need to turn our thinking around.

We often create health problems by engaging in poor eating habits and a lifestyle of body neglect. Sometimes we eat the right food, but the food itself is deficient. To correct this problem, it may be necessary to take supplements in pill form. There is, however, *no substitute* for the basic nourishment that God has created to fortify our bodies against disease.

VITAMINS

What is your vitamin IQ? List the names of at least five vitamins. (Some researchers list twenty different vitamins.)

1. _____

2. _____

3. _____

4. _____

5. _____

(If you can't think of any vitamins, think of the letters of the alphabet and try again.)

Taber's Cyclopedic Medical Dictionary states, "Vitamins are any of a group of organic substances other than protein, carbohydrates, fats, minerals and organic salts which are essential for normal metabolism, growth, and development of the body."[2] Vitamins retain their original form in the body and act as coenzymes to bring about changes and processes within the body's cells. Vitamins help regulate the function of the body's processes. The presence or absence of vitamins in very small amounts means the difference between good and poor health.

The green leaves of plants are the laboratories in which plant vitamins are manufactured. Seeds (such as beans, peas, kernels of wheat and corn) also contain vitamins that the plant has provided to nourish the next generation of plants. The lean meat of animals contains vitamins; the organs (such as the heart or liver) contain even more vitamins because the animal's digestive system has stored them there. The yolks of eggs contain the vitamins that the mother animals have provided for their young.

Vitamins in fruits and vegetables are called water soluble, since they can be dissolved in water. Those found in liver and eggs are fat soluble.[3]

Check your vitamin IQ list with the following list. Vitamins we know the most about are called by a letter and also by a chemical name.[4]

> Vitamin A (carotene)
> B complex: B_1 (thiamine), B_2 (riboflavin), B_6 (pyridoxine), B_{12} (cyanocobalamine), biotin, choline, folic acid, inositol, niacin, para-aminobenzoic acid (PABA), pantothenic acid

Some researchers list:

> Vitamin B_{15} (pangamic acid)
> Vitamin B_{17} (amygdalin)
> Vitamin C (ascorbic acid)
> Vitamin D (D-2, D-3, D-4, D-5)
> Vitamin E (tocopheral)
> Vitamin K (menadione)

Some researchers also list:

> Vitamin F (unsaturated fatty acids)
> Vitamin P (bioflavinoids)

Let us go on an imaginary shopping trip. Place a check mark next to the items on the following list you *seldom* or *never* eat. We won't need to purchase these.

RICH SOURCES OF NUTRIENTS[5]

VITAMIN A

Liver
Egg yolks
Yellow fruits and vegetables (such as carrots)
Dark-green fruits and vegetables (such as spinach)
Whole milk and milk products
Cod-liver oil

VITAMIN B$_1$

Brewer's yeast
Whole grains
Blackstrap molasses
Brown rice
Organ meats
Meats, fish, and poultry
Egg yolks
Legumes
Nuts
Wheat germ
Sunflower seeds

VITAMIN B$_2$

Brewer's yeast
Fruit
Whole grains
Milk
Blackstrap molasses
Fish
Organ meats
Poultry
Egg yolks
Legumes
Nuts (except almonds)
Green leafy vegetables

VITAMIN B$_6$

Meat
Rice
Whole grains
Organ meats
Brewer's yeast
Blackstrap molasses
Walnuts
Wheat germ
Bran
Legumes
Avocados
Bananas
Cabbage
Prunes
Raisins
Blueberries
Green leafy vegetables
Desiccated liver
Trout

VITAMIN B$_{12}$

Organ meats
Fish and beef
Eggs
Cottage cheese
Cheese
Milk and milk products
Trout

BIOTIN

Egg yolks
Liver
Unpolished rice
Brewer's yeast
Whole grains
Sardines
Legumes

CHOLINE

Egg yolks
Organ meats
Brewer's yeast
Wheat germ
Soybeans
Fish
Legumes
Lecithin

FOLIC ACID

Dark-green leafy vegetables
Organ meats
Lean beef and veal
Brewer's yeast
Root vegetables
Wheat cereals
Whole grains
Spinach
Salmon
Milk
Eggs

INOSITOL

Whole grains
Citrus fruits (such as oranges)
Brewer's yeast
Molasses
Meat
Milk
Nuts
Vegetables
Lecithin
Organ meats

Some researchers list:
B_{17} AMYGDALIN

Whole kernels of apricots, apples,
cherries, peaches, and plums

NIACIN

Lean meats
Poultry and fish
Brewer's yeast
Peanuts
Eggs
Whole grains
Milk and milk products
Rice bran
Desiccated liver

PARA-AMINOBENZOIC ACID

Bran
Organ meats
Milk
Wheat germ
Yogurt

Some researchers list:
B_{15} PANGAMIC ACID

Brewer's yeast
Whole grains
Brown rice
Sunflower, pumpkin, and sesame
seeds
Organ meats

PANTOTHENIC ACID

Organ meats
Brewer's yeast
Egg yolks
Legumes
Whole grains
Wheat germ
Mushrooms
Salmon
Liver

VITAMIN C

Onions
Citrus fruits (such as oranges)
Apples
Rose hips
Pears
Acerola cherries
Apricots
Alfalfa seeds, sprouted
Peaches
Cantaloupe
Plums
Pineapple
Strawberries
Carrots
Broccoli
Lettuce
Tomatoes
Celery
Green peppers
Cabbage
Radishes

VITAMIN D

Salmon
Sardines
Herring
Eggs
Molasses
Brown rice
Green leafy vegetables
Brewer's yeast
Vitamin D–fortified milk and milk
    products
Egg yolks
Organ meats
Cod-liver oil
Bone meal
Sunlight

VITAMIN E

Cold pressed oils
Eggs
Wheat germ
Organ meats
Brown rice
Molasses
Sweet potatoes
Leafy vegetables
Desiccated liver
Fruits
Nuts (such as almonds)

VITAMIN F

Vegetable oils
Butter
Sunflower seeds
Wheat germ

VITAMIN K

Wheat, rye, alfalfa
Green leafy vegetables
Egg yolks
Safflower oil
Blackstrap molasses
Liver
Cauliflower
Soybeans
Oatmeal

P BIOFLAVINOIDS

Lemon and grapefruit
Citrus fruits
Grapes
Apricots
Black currants
Cherries
Buckwheat
Plums

Go back over your list and note any vitamin category where you have several check marks and list those vitamins:

1. _____

2. _____

3. _____

There is a good chance that you may be lacking these vitamins in your system. Many other foods, too numerous to mention, also contain these nutrients. Refer to the reference section for additional reading material on this subject.

Can specific health problems be caused by not getting an adequate amount of vitamins? Yes. *Taber's Cyclopedic Medical Dictionary* describes avitaminosis as a disease due to lack of vitamins in the diet—a deficiency disease. Listed among specific deficiency disorders are the following:[6]

Vitamin-A deficiency—reduced resistance to infections, night blindness, impaired growth, and poor development in children.

Vitamin-B deficiency—beriberi, pellagra, digestive disturbances, nervous disorders, problems with the heart, liver, spleen, kidneys, pancreas, thyroid, adrenals, pituitary, and salivary glands.

Vitamin-C deficiency—scurvy, defective teeth, pyorrhea, anorexia (loss of appetite), anemia, malnutrition, injury to bone, cells, and blood vessels.

Vitamin-D deficiency—imperfect skeletal formation, bone disease, rickets, dental caries.

Vitamin-K deficiency—delayed blood clotting and hemorrhaging.

Dr. Wilfred E. Shute's *Vitamin E Book* states vitamin E affects the cardiovascular and circulatory systems. He also believes vitamin E reduces the oxygen requirements of the tissues and cells and helps form new skin.[7]

Research proves severe vitamin deficiencies can cause major illnesses. It may be possible that *minor* vitamin deficiencies over a period of time could also cause illnesses.

Thirty-year-old Anita, mother of two, came into my office complaining of night blindness. She said her 11:00 PM to 7:00 AM shift at her job necessitated driving at night. As she told me how she had nearly caused a serious highway accident on a dark, rainy night, her panic was obvious. She said her eye doctor reported that her eyesight was good. When questioned about her diet, she said, "I don't eat right. I am too busy to prepare nutritious meals." She recognized her problem, but didn't know how to solve it. I reviewed the dietary questionnaire she had filled out and noticed foods rich in vitamin A were scarce. "It's vitamin A that you need," I said.

I requested she make out menus including an overabundance of vitamin A foods on her shopping list. On the top of her list were dark green, leafy, and yellow vegetables and fruits. I told her broccoli, carrots, liver, spinach, eggs, and cheese were especially high in vitamin A. Because of special tests I had run, I suggested she take 10,000 IU of vitamin A once a day, B complex, vitamins C and E, plus calcium, magnesium, and zinc.

After two months on this regimen, she began to notice a change. After six months her night vision improved so that she could even see when it was dark and raining. Her night vision is not yet perfect, but she is able to drive herself safely to work.

How is it possible that people become vitamin deficient in today's world of advanced technology? To answer that question, let us examine the way food is prepared and preserved in our society.

Commercial canning destroys 50–80 percent of the vitamin C in peas, lima beans, spinach, and asparagus. Freshly prepared applesauce retains only 20–30 percent of the vitamin C value of the apple. Pickling, salting, curing, or fermenting usually causes complete loss of vitamin C. Pasteurization causes a loss of from 30–60 percent of vitamin C.[8]

Dr. Wilfred Shute says, "Eighty-seven percent of vitamin E is lost in milling by removing the germ from wheat; the remainder is lost in the bleaching process." According to Shute, vitamin E has also been almost completely removed from refined, hydrogenated oils, soy and cottonseed margarines, and mayonnaise.[9]

The B vitamins are lost when the wheat germ and the outer layer of grains are removed in the milling process for white flour. Some, *but not all,* of the essential nutrients lost in the milling process are added when flour or cereals are labeled "enriched." Whole-grain foods are much better than refined products. Beriberi, a disease resulting from a deficiency of B1 (thiamine), is common in parts of Asia where polished rice forms the staple food. Ironically, the treatment for beriberi is medicine made from rice polishings that contain the thiamine-rich seed coat.

High temperatures destroy B vitamins. The losses of B6 and pantothenic acid can be 91 percent in canned foods.

Are you beginning to see how a steady diet of refined, processed, and canned foods could cause vitamin deficiencies?

Fresh fruits and vegetables that are high quality and not stored long are best. If the quality of the fresh food is poor, or you can't shop frequently, frozen food would be next best. Blanching of vegetables and fruits before freezing may cause some loss of vitamin C and B1 (thiamine). Frozen meat, fish, and poultry compare in vitamin content with fresh if they are wrapped well and properly frozen.

Vitamin A and D are lost when fat is removed from milk. Margarine is also deficient in these vitamins. These products may be fortified, but labels don't tell how much.

A significant loss of vitamins can occur during food preparation and cooking. Vegetables shouldn't be soaked or cooked for long periods of time. Steaming or cooking in a pressure cooker or microwave with very little water, and only until the vegetables are still crunchy, preserves the most vitamins. Baking vegetables whole is another excellent method for preserving vitamins. Boiling vegetables in water and cooking them until mushy causes the highest nutrient loss.

MINERALS

Vitamins have been center stage for a decade or more. Everyone reads and hears about their importance in the diet. But minerals are taken for granted. The assumption is that since minerals aren't lost easily in food preparation, the supply is adequate for the body. Dr. Harry Warren, professor of geology at the University of British Columbia, Vancouver, says minerals in soil and water have a far greater effect on health than climate. He feels it is possible that physiological effects of the mineral content of the soil are retarded birthrate, goiter, anemia, and poor digestion.[10]

Taber's Cyclopedic Medical Dictionary defines *mineral* as an inorganic element or compound occurring in nature. Minerals are essential constituents of all cells. They form the greater portion of bone, teeth, and nails, and are essential components of the respiratory pigments, enzymes, and enzyme systems.[11]

Because mineral salts and water are excreted daily from the body, they must be replaced through food intake. Dr. F. P. Anita, in his book *Clinical Dietetics and Nutrition,* says, "The body can tolerate a deficiency of vitamins for a longer period of time than a deficiency of minerals. A slight change in the blood concentration of important minerals may rapidly endanger life."[12]

Your mineral intake depends on what you ingest, how it is prepared, and *how and where it was grown*. Plants grown in the Great Lakes region and the Pacific Northwest (two goiter belts) are deficient in iodine. Iron-deficient soils have been reported in most of the fifty states, especially in Florida and Massachusetts, parts of Utah, western Colorado, the Salt River Valley of Arizona, the Imperial Valley of California (the greatest fruit growing area in America), the Snake River Valley in Idaho, central Washington, and the lower Rio Grande Valley in Texas.[13]

There are two groups of minerals essential to life. The major minerals, also called "macrominerals," are required in a greater amount than the trace minerals, or microminerals. Both categories must be present in the right ratio for good health.

How much do you know about minerals? Can you list any of the seven major macrominerals?

1. _____

2. _____

3. _____

4. _____

5. _____

6. _____

7. _____

There are nine trace or microminerals. Can you list any?

1. _____

2. _____

3. _____

4. _____

5. _____

6. _____

7. _____

8. _____

9. _____

If you failed to name any, read on and then fill in the blanks.

MACROMINERALS

Calcium
Magnesium
Phosphorous
Sodium

Potassium
Chloride
Sulfur

MICROMINERALS

Iron
Zinc
Selenium
Manganese
Molybdenum

Copper
Fluorine
Iodine
Chromium

Other trace minerals are being studied at the present time. It has been shown that some of the trace elements are important in animal nutrition, but more research is needed with human beings.

Before we make a trip to the grocery store to shop for high-mineral foods we need a shopping list. Read over the following list, and place a check mark beside the ones you never eat. You won't need to purchase these.

HIGH MINERAL FOOD[14]

MACROMINERALS

CALCIUM

Milk and milk products
Liver
Green leafy vegetables
Canned salmon
Molasses
Citrus fruits
Bone meal
Legumes
Dolomite

Yogurt
Almonds

MAGNESIUM

Seafood
Whole grains
Honey
Spinach
Kelp
Tuna

Dark-green vegetables
Molasses
Nuts
Almonds
Bone meal
Bran
Soybeans

PHOSPHORUS

Fish, meats, poultry
Eggs
Legumes
Milk and milk products
Nuts
Whole-grain cereals
Bone meal

SODIUM

Seafood
Table salt
Baking powder and baking soda

POTASSIUM

Bananas
Lean meats
Orange juice
Whole grains
Potatoes

MICROMINERALS

IRON

Liver
Organ meats
Shredded wheat
Egg yolks
Fish and poultry
Whole-grain cereals
Blackstrap molasses

Vegetables
Dried fruits
Peaches
Legumes
Peanut butter
Sunflower seeds
Bran
Hominy

CHLORIDE

Table salt
Seafood
Meats
Ripe olives
Rye flour

SULFUR

Fish
Beef
Wheat germ
Eggs
Meats
Cabbage
Lean meats
Brussels sprouts
Celery
Processed foods
Milk products
Kelp

Cherry juice
Dried peas and beans
Green leafy vegetables
Dried fruits
Desiccated liver
Wheat germ

ZINC

Liver

Sunflower seeds
Eggs
Seafood
Organ meats
Mushrooms
Brewer's yeast
Soybeans
Poultry
Milk
Whole grains

SELENIUM

Tuna
Meat
Brewer's yeast
Wheat germ and bran
Chicken
Broccoli
Whole grains
Egg yolks
Brown rice
Milk
Garlic
Green peppers
Pineapples
Pears
Bananas

MOLYBDENUM

Legumes
Whole-grain cereals
Milk
Liver
Dark-green vegetables

COPPER

Organ meats
Soybeans

Seafood
Nuts
Avocado
Legumes
Molasses
Corn oil margarine
Raisins
Bone meal
Liver

CHROMIUM

Meat
Corn oil
Cheese
Whole-grain cereals
Dried beans
Brewer's yeast

IODINE

Seafood
Salt-water fish
Kelp
Sea salt
Iodized salt

MANGANESE

Bran
Whole grains
Green leafy vegetables
Legumes
Eggplant
Nuts

FLUORINE

Tea
Seafood
Fluoridated water
Bone meal

Go back and note any mineral category where you have placed several check marks.

1. _____

2. _____

3. _____

4. _____

5. _____

6. _____

Is it possible you could be deficient in these minerals? Other foods high in minerals are listed in the resources for further reading found in the reference section.

Let us take a look at some of the problems associated with mineral deficiencies.

MACROMINERALS[15]

Calcium deficiency—Rickets, osteoporosis, heart palpitations, insomnia, muscle cramps, nervousness, tooth decay, arm and leg numbness, brittle fingernails.

Magnesium deficiency—Tremors, rapid pulse, confusion, easily aroused anger, disorientation.

Phosphorous deficiency—Fatigue, appetite loss, irregular breathing, nervous disorders, overweight, and weight loss.

Chlorine deficiency—Hair and tooth loss, poor muscular contraction and impaired digestion.

Sulfur deficiency—No known symptoms.

Potassium deficiency—Dry skin, edema, insomnia, muscle damage, slow and irregular heartbeat, nervousness, anxiety, aching muscles.

Sodium deficiency—Cramps, intestinal gas, vomiting, appetite loss, eye disturbances.

MICROMINERALS

Iron deficiency—Iron deficiency anemia, fatigue, constipation, breathing difficulties, brittle nails, sore inflamed tongue.

Zinc deficiency—Loss of taste, fatigue, poor appetite, retarded growth, sterility, prolonged wound healing, delayed sexual maturity.

Selenium deficiency—Peroxidation of fats, blood hemolytic problems, mercury toxicity, pancreatic insufficiency, cardiac toxicity of drugs, aging pigment.

Manganese deficiency—Ear noises, loss of hearing, dizziness, muscle coordination failure.

Molybdenum deficiency—No known symptoms.

Chromium deficiency—Glucose intolerance in diabetics, disturbed amino acid metabolism, atherosclerosis.

Iodine deficiency—Cold hands and feet, dry hair, irritability, nervousness, obesity.

Flourine deficiency—Tooth decay.

Copper deficiency—Anemia, atherosclerosis, baldness.

The danger of listing vitamin and mineral deficiency symptoms in a book is that readers will use them to attempt self-diagnosis. Don't run to the health food store or drug store and try to treat yourself. Only a trained clinician knows how to do this. Your job is to increase the intake of food rich in the nutrients you seem to lack.

List those foods you know you should increase in your daily diet. Use a separate sheet of paper if necessary.

1. _____

2. _____

3. _____

4. _____

5. _____

6. _____

7. _____

Are you experiencing problems with your health that might be connected with inadequate intake or poor assimilation of some vitamins and minerals?

ENZYMES

Before we discuss enzymes, you need to realize that the study of enzymes is very technical and would require more than one chapter. This book will only acquaint you with them. Enzymes are organic catalysts produced by living cells, but they can act independently. They are complex *proteins* capable of inducing chemical changes *in other substances* without being changed themselves in the process.[16]

Next to hormones and other active substances, body enzymes have a major role. In a variety of reactions they *direct, accelerate, modify,* or *retard all body functions.*[17]

I like to think of enzymes as a unit and call enzymes the conductor of the personal body orchestra. As long as the conductor is functioning well the orchestra sounds good. If he breaks his arm, gets sick, or loses his hearing, the orchestra suffers and will not function properly. Enzymes cause reactions, speed them up, slow them down, or change them. As you may have guessed, enzymes are a key to life itself. Each enzyme is essential. If one is absent or present in an insufficient amount, there will be trouble or functional failure of the cells or tissue involved. An example of enzyme function other than in the human body is seen in the manufacture of cheese and vinegar.

In the nineteenth century Louis Pasteur proved that the microorganisms in yeast contain ferments or enzymes and can cause chemical reactions.

In our own time enzyme research regarding the function of the human body is a growing field. There is much to be discovered. It is believed that almost all physiological reactions

Site	Secretion	Enzyme	Substrate	Degree of Digestion	Products of Digestion
Mouth	Saliva	Pytalin	Starch	Slight	Dextrins, maltose
		Maltase	Maltose	Very slight	Glucose
Stomach	Gastric juice	Pepsin	Protein	Incomplete	Preteoses, peptones
		Rennin	Casein	Nearly complete	Paracasein
		Lipase	Emulsified fats	Very slight	Fatty acids, glycerol
Intestine	Pancreatic juice	Trypsin	Proteins		
		Chymo-trypsin	Proteoses	Nearly complete	Amino acids
		Carboxy-peptidase	Peptones Peptides		
		Steapsin	Fats	Nearly complete	Insoluble fatty acids, glycerol
		Amylopsin	Starch	Nearly complete	Dextrins, maltose
Intestine	Intestinal juice and intestinal mucosa	Erepsin	Ordinary peptides	Nearly complete	Amino acids
		Amylase	Starch	Nearly complete	Dextrins, maltose
		Enterokinase	Trypsinogen		Trypsin
		Maltase	Maltose	Complete	Glucose
		Lactase	Lactose	Complete	Glucose, galactose
		Sucrase	Sucrose	Usually complete	Glucose, fructose
		Nucleosidases (in mucosa)	Nucleosides	Usually complete	Purine bases, carbo-hydrates

Adapted from H. C. Biddle and V. W. Floutz, *Chemistry in Health and Disease*, 6th ed. (Philadelphia: F. A. Davis, 1965).

like muscle contraction, nerve conduction, and urine excretion are conditioned by enzyme activities.

Examine the chart carefully so we can discuss the action

of enzymes in the body.

More than 650 enzymes are known to exist. The chemical reactions necessary for proper body functions are dependent upon enzymes. There are fat-, protein-, starch-, and sugar-splitting enzymes. Another enzyme causes coagulation of the blood.

Sometimes enzymes require coenzymes to activate them. Hydrochloric acid, for example, is necessary for the enzyme pepsin to become active. Vitamins are coenzymes and have to be present in the correct amount for enough enzymes to be formed to carry out many vital body reactions.[19]

Now that you understand the importance of enzymes, let us look at a specific example: food digestion. It is one of the most obvious enzymatic reactions in the body. If your food gives you gas, pain, belching, and burning, something is wrong. The causes of indigestion are not always easy to determine, and a medical doctor should be consulted if the condition persists. But there is a simple remedy you can try that won't hurt you. You may take digestive enzymes containing the enzymes, papain, pepsin, and hydrochloric acid.

A college student was brought to me by his mother. One of her complaints was *his* habit of belching. When questioned, he said that he often had indigestion. I suggested he might benefit by taking a digestive enzyme with each meal. One week later his mother called me and said he had completely stopped belching, and he told her he felt much better. She laughingly said, "We aren't even afraid anymore to let him go out in public." She went on to say, "Now, I have a different problem, since he can digest pizza, he wants it every meal."

Proteolytic enzymes dissolve protein. Two common examples of these enzymes are bromelin in raw pineapple and papain in raw papaya. Enzymes are heat sensitive, and cooking or canning these fruits will destroy the enzymes. Have you ever questioned why the directions on the Jell-O box caution not to add *fresh* pineapple but canned is acceptable? The proteolytic enzymes in fresh pineapple dissolve the protein in Jell-O and it won't gel. When pineapple is heated for canning, its enzymes are destroyed. Another example is meat tenderizer made of papain

BLUEPRINT FOR HEALTH

(papaya). It breaks down the protein structure and tenderizes the meat.

Since we know that heat destroys enzymes in food, we should realize the necessity of eating raw fruits and vegetables each day to provide enzymes for better body function.

FIBER

Why the fiber craze? David Reuben in his book *The Save Your Life Diet* said, "Fiber is the most exciting medical story in the 1970's."[20] He believes that by adding the missing roughage to our daily diet we provide protection against the following conditions:

1. Cancer of the colon and rectum.
2. Ischemic heart disease.
3. Diverticular disease of the colon.
4. Appendicitis.
5. Phlebitis and resulting blood clots to the lungs.
6. Obesity.[21]

Fiber, known to our ancestors as roughage, was recommended for the diet about 1920 by Dr. John Harvy Kellogg, of the Michigan cereal family, while he was medical director of a sanitorium in Battle Creek. The diet he favored for his patients was potatoes, dates, carrots, wheat, bran, nuts, and steel-cut Scotch oats. He also felt fruits, cereals, and fresh vegetables should be included in every American's diet.[22]

Some high-fiber foods are apples, peaches, cooked asparagus, cooked beans, whole-grain breads and cereals (such as oatmeal), 100% All Bran, miller's bran, sweet corn, dried figs and prunes, lentils, cooked peas, potatoes, whole-grain rice, raspberries, blackberries, strawberries, tomatoes, zucchini, eggplant, brussels sprouts, cabbage, and carrots.[23]

Make a list of the high-fiber foods you eat. Remember breads and cereals must be whole grain or they don't count.

1. _____

2. _____

3. _____

4. _____

5. _____

6. _____

7. _____

Are you constipated? Fiber acts as a sponge to draw water into the large intestines and makes the feces larger, softer, and easier to pass.

British physician, Dr. Denis Burkett, believes that lack of fiber allows cancer-causing substances to reside in the gut too long. He recommends fiber be increased in the average daily diet.

Obesity is rare in countries where large amounts of starchy carbohydrates are eaten complete with their natural fiber. Fiber itself has few, if any calories. It absorbs water as it passes through your digestive tract. It is filling, and you are more likely to feel satisfied from a high-fiber meal.[24]

A study conducted at the Veterans Administration Hospital in Lexington, Kentucky, suggests long-term, high-fiber diets can reduce harmful low-density lipoproteins (LDL) and increase beneficial high-density lipoproteins (HDL). These changes may lessen the risk of heart disease.

Endocrinologist Dr. James W. Anderson has even developed high-fiber diets for diabetics. He has proven that after a high-fiber meal the diabetic's blood sugar isn't as high as after one low in fiber.[25]

When you start eating a high-fiber diet, you must remember to drink lots of water and liquids. You must also make sure your nutrient intake is adequate. An increase in fiber of the poorly nourished, like adolescents or the elderly, could cause further depletion of calcium, zinc, iron, magnesium, phosphorus, and copper. Nutrient intake should be increased before fiber is added.

Do you need to increase your fiber intake? Refer to the fiber chart and list the fiber foods you like below.

1. _____

2. _____

3. _____

4. _____

5. _____

6. _____

GUIDE TO FIBER IN FOODS
James Anderson, M.D.

Food	Serving size	Grams/ serving	Calories/ serving	Fiber, in grams/ serving[26]
Apple, fresh	½ large	83	42	2.0
Apple, cooked	½ large	83	40	2.0
Apricots, fresh	2	72	32	1.4
Asparagus, cooked	½ cup	93	18	3.5
Banana, fresh	½ medium	54	48	1.5
Bean sprouts, fresh	½ cup	58	13	1.5
Beans, brown, cooked	½ cup	84	80	8.4
Beans, green, cooked	½ cup	64	10	2.1
Beans, kidney, cooked	½ cup	93	94	9.7
Beans, lima, cooked	½ cup	85	63	8.3
Beans, pinto, cooked	½ cup	84	78	8.9
Beans, white, cooked	½ cup	90	79	7.9
Beets, cooked	½ cup	85	33	2.1
Blackberries, fresh	¾ cup	108	40	6.7
Bread, pumpernickel	¾ slice	24	58	1.4
corn bread	1 square	30	58	1.1

Food	Serving size	Grams/serving	Calories/serving	Fiber, in grams/serving[26]
French	1 slice	25	71	0.7
rye	1 slice	25	62	0.8
white	1 slice	25	64	0.7
whole meal	1 slice	25	56	2.1
whole wheat	1 slice	25	59	1.3
Broccoli, cooked	½ cup	93	18	3.5
Brussels sprouts, cooked	½ cup	78	20	2.3
Cabbage, white, cooked	½ cup	85	10	2.1
Carrots, raw	½ cup	55	15	1.8
Cauliflower, cooked	½ cup	90	14	1.6
Celery, raw	½ cup	60	8	1.1
Cereal, All Bran® (100%)	⅓ cup	28	70	8.4
Bran Chex®	½ cup	21	67	4.1
Corn Chex®	¾ cup	21	71	2.6
Corn Bran®	½ cup	21	68	4.4
Corn Flakes®	¾ cup	21	70	2.6
Grapenut Flakes®	⅔ cup	21	71	2.5
Grapenuts®	3 tbs	21	70	2.7
Oat Bran®, dry	¼ cup	20	58	5.3
Oat Flakes	½ cup	21	72	2.5
Oatmeal, instant dry	¾ pkg	21	74	2.5
Oats, whole dry	¼ cup	21	71	2.9
Post Toasties®	1 cup	21	71	2.6
Puffed Wheat®	¾ cup	21	68	3.4
Ralston® dry	3 tbs	21	72	2.1
Shredded Wheat®	1 biscuit	21	70	2.8
Total®	¾ cup	21	75	2.5
Wheaties®	¾ cup	14	73	2.6
Cherries, fresh	10 large	68	38	1.1
Corn, sweet, fresh	½ med. ear	63	72	2.6
Cornmeal, fine	2 tbs	17	57	1.6
Cracker, graham	2 squares	14	53	1.4
rye wafer	3 wafers	20	64	2.3
saltine	6 crackers	20	76	0.8
Cranberries, raw	½ cup	96	31	4.0
Cucumber, raw	½ cup	70	6	1.1
Eggplant, raw	½ cup	100	16	2.5
Figs, dried	1 medium	20	46	3.7
Flour, rye, dark	2½ tbs	20	63	2.5
rye, light	2½ tbs	16	56	0.5

Food	Serving size	Grams/ serving	Calories/ serving	Fiber, in grams/ serving[26]
self-raising	2½ tbs	18	61	0.7
wheat, white	2½ tbs	18	62	0.5
wheat, whole meal	2½ tbs	19	60	1.8
wheat, whole wheat	2½ tbs	19	62	1.4
Grapefruit, fresh	½	87	31	0.8
Grapes, black fresh	15	60	45	0.5
Grapes, white fresh	10	50	36	0.5
Kale, cooked	½ cup	65	15	1.3
Lentils, cooked	½ cup	100	97	3.7
Lettuce, fresh	1 cup	55	5	0.8
Macaroni, cooked	½ cup	70	77	0.6
Melon, cantaloupe	1 cup	160	39	1.6
honeydew	1 cup	170	42	1.5
watermelon	1 cup	160	35	1.4
Mushrooms, raw	½ cup	35	7	0.9
Mustard greens, raw	1 cup	55	7	2.0
Nectarine, raw	1 small	69	44	1.5
Nuts, almonds, whole	1 tbs	8	46	1.1
chestnuts	3	26	46	1.8
peanuts, roasted	1 tbs	9	52	0.8
pecans	1 tbs	7.5	49	0.5
Okra, raw	½ cup	50	13	1.6
Onion, raw	½ cup	58	14	1.2
Orange, fresh	1 small	78	35	1.6
Peach, fresh	1 medium	100	38	2.3
Pear, fresh	½ medium	82	44	2.0
Peas, canned, cooked	½ cup	85	63	6.7
Pepper, green, raw	½ cup	58	10	1.1
Pineapple, fresh	½ cup	78	41	0.8
Plum, fresh	3 small	85	38	1.8
Popcorn, popped	3 cups	18	62	3.0
Potato, sweet, cooked	½ medium	75	79	2.1
Potato, white, baked	½ medium	75	72	1.9
Prunes, dried	2	15	38	2.8
Radishes, raw	½ cup	58	7	1.3
Raisins, dried	1½ tbs	14	39	1.0
Raspberries, red, fresh	1 cup	124	42	9.2
Rice, brown, cooked	⅓ cup	65	72	1.6
Rice, white, cooked	⅓ cup	68	76	0.5
Roll, dinner	¾ roll	20	60	0.6

Food	Serving size	Grams/ serving	Calories/ serving	Fiber, in grams/ serving[26]
Roll, whole wheat	¾ roll	21	55	1.2
Spaghetti, cooked	½ cup	70	76	0.8
Spinach, fresh	1 cup	55	8	0.2
Squash, summer, cooked	½ cup	90	8	2.0
Squash, winter, cooked	1 cup	240	82	7.0
Strawberries, fresh	1 cup	143	45	3.1
Tangerine, fresh	1 large	101	39	2.0
Tomato, cooked	½ cup	121	20	1.5
Tomato, raw	1 small	100	18	1.5
Turnip, cooked	½ cup	93	12	2.0
Yam, cooked	⅓ cup	66	72	2.6
Zucchini, raw	½ cup	65	7	2.0

James W. Anderson, M.D., *Diabetes* (New York: Arco Publishing, 1981), 141-43. Used by permission.

BLUEPRINT FOR HEALTH

9   MODERN-DAY FOODS—JUNK OR JEWELS?

Agriculture revolution. Agri-business. Mechanical agriculture. Chemical farmer. Degenerative farm. Organic farm. Regenerative farm. These are just some of the terms used to identify modern farming operations.[1]

Since the forties, when I grew up on a farm in Indiana, farming has undergone a metamorphosis. We had our own chickens, cows, and pigs; fruits and vegetables came from the garden; and wheat, corn, oats, soybeans, and alfalfa grew in the fields. There was no danger of going hungry when we were surrounded by all that food.

My family is still in farming, but now it is big business. Some call it agri-business. The cows, chickens, and pigs are gone. Although the garden is still there, the crops are limited to one or two, such as corn, beans, or wheat, and the acreage has increased from hundreds to thousands of acres.

The modern farm is set up for mass food production, and farming has become a highly competitive business. To get top yields, chemical fertilizers are applied to the ground and plants. The heavy workload of farming hundreds of acres to produce crops in a short time has led to the use of strong pesticides, herbicides, and chemical fertilizers.

Science and technology have brought about many changes—some good, some bad. Because of cheaper, more abundant food production, we can help feed starving people in other nations, though I wonder if the chemicals and pesticides used on the crops and the antibiotics fed to animals might have dangerously adulterated our food supply. At the same time, degenerative diseases are increasing. Could there be any connection?

Aldo Leopold sums up my thoughts: "We abuse land because we regard it as a *commodity* belonging to us. When we see land as a *community* to which we belong, we may begin to use it with love and respect. There is no other way for land to survive the impact of mechanized man, nor for us to reap from it the aesthetic harvest it is capable, under science, of contributing to culture."[2]

Paul and Dale Billberg of Wannaska, Minnesota, have learned to love and respect their land. Many years ago they were alarmed when the harvest from their 1500-acre grain and livestock farm began to shrink. A number of sheep and lambs were diseased. Their soil was becoming harder, and the fertile tilled land was eroding at an alarming rate. They wondered whether the agricultural chemicals applied to their soil might be sapping this precious resource of its vigor. So they embarked on a program of "organic farming." For three years they had above-average crops, but when the soil had depleted its nutrients the crops suffered. It took two years of rotating nitrogen-producing legumes with nitrogen-depleting crops, such as corn, to return productivity to normal. The Billbergs have livestock, and spread nutrient-rich animal manure over their fields. Dale says, "We are soil builders. If the soil is healthy, the crops it nourishes will be healthy." She says they feel better about farming now and are more conscious of their responsibilities as stewards of the land.[3]

Robert Rodale, publisher of *Organic Farming* and *The New Farm* magazine, runs his own agriculture research center, a 320-acre farm and largely organic integrated-crop and finishing operation in Kutztown, Pennsylvania. In 1983 he gathered his extensive data and compared his regenerative farm's performance with local and national standards. The results were impressive. His organization actively supported the Agricultural Productivity Act of 1983, which provides for similar studies of regenerative farms throughout the nation.[4]

The late Dr. Carey Reams, a biochemist and biophysicist, states, "Our health is dependent upon the soil. We've got to start working with our soil to improve the quality of the fruits, vegetables, grains, and foods we eat."[5]

Science and technology have opened up wide horizons. Many life-changing achievements have been made, and the food industry has been influenced by these discoveries. God created the human body and the food to nourish it. As Christians, we need to ask ourselves if we are well-informed about the food we put into our wonderfully designed bodies.

Is the quality of our food what we believe it to be? Biochemist Ross Hume Hall believes it is not. He says the farmer provides the raw material to the food technologists who manipulate it and manufacture it into products. For instance, wheat has always been partially refined, but now the wheat germ is lost because of the heat of the high-speed rollers used to process the grain. Also, the bran and the accessory factors (such as minerals and vitamins) are discarded early in the refining process (see figure 9.1).

Food engineers lose sight of the raw material and think of it in terms of carbohydrate (starch, sugar), protein (amino acids), and fat (oil). They tend to see what can be fabricated out of these components, such as textured vegetable proteins and chemically modified food starches. These starches are used in baby food, pie filling, creamed butter sauces, cheese sauces, and gravies, to which the chemists also add artificial colors, flavors, preservatives.[6] Then the advertising firms promote the product.

Do you believe food advertising is always truthful? I remember one television commercial for "Trix" breakfast cereal. The ad sang out, "There's lemon, there's orange in every bite," and the word "fruit" was repeated often. But the real contents of "Trix" are only fruit flavors, citric acid, and 35.9 percent sugar and other assorted ingredients—*no fruit*.

As you watch television think about the food ads, and see if you have been misled by any of them. List your discoveries here:

1. _____

2. _____

3. _____

4. _____

Step back with me to the year 1900 for a day at my great-grandparents' house. All of the meals were home cooked.

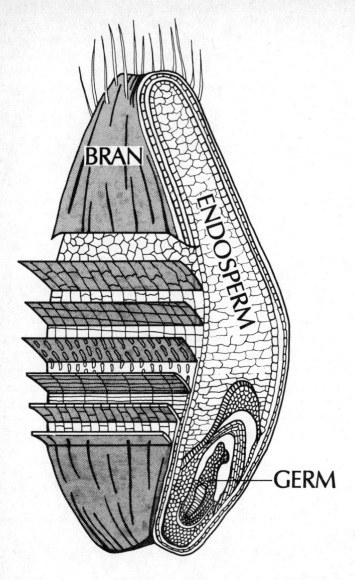

Fig 9.1 A grain of wheat. (Adapted by Louise Bauer from the Kansas Wheat Commission)

Restaurants weren't a way of life then. The menus included fresh vegetables and fruit in the summer, fresh eggs, fresh milk, potatoes, cereal grains, and small amounts of meat, poultry, and fish. In the winter, vegetables and fruits were home canned. Homemade whole-wheat bread was a highlight of the meal. The dessert was pie, cake, bread pudding, or custard—all made at home. The choice of drinks were coffee, tea, or milk.

My great-grandmother spent a lot of time preparing wholesome meals. Since nothing was processed or packaged in those days, the food was free of artificial chemicals. Great-grandmother had control over the food she served and a thorough knowledge of its sources. She grew it, prepared it, preserved it, and served it. It was close to its natural state.

But there were problems with the diet in those days as well. It was high in saturated fats such as lard, butter, cheese, ham, and fat. Vegetables were often overcooked, and salads were not popular. The science of nutrition was almost nonexistent.

In great-grandmother's time the major killer diseases were tuberculosis, gastroenteritis, diphtheria, poliomyelitis, influenza, and pneumonia. In recent years, with the discovery of new drugs, the incidence of these infectious diseases has decreased.

The chart on page 98 released by the U.S. Department of Health and Welfare, National Center for Health Statistics shows a comparison of the major killer diseases between 1900–1977.[7]

Michael Jacobson, Ph.D., head of the Center for Science in the Public Interest, reports that the most important changes in the American diet in the last sixty-five years have been:

- *The increase in fat consumption.* Fat provided *42 percent* of our calories in 1976, which is a 31 percent increase over the *32 percent* of our calories that fat supplied in 1910.
- *The decrease in* complex *carbohydrates (basically starch) consumption.* In 1976, only *21 percent* of our calories were complex carbohydrates, which is *43 percent* less than the *37 percent* of calories in 1909–1913.
- *The increase in sweetener consumption.* Refined sugar, corn syrup, and other caloric sweeteners supplied *18 percent* of

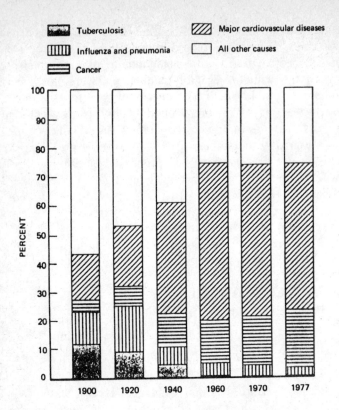

Fig 9.2 Deaths for selected causes as a percent of all deaths: United States, selected years, 1900–1977. (Source: National Center for Health Statistics, Division of Vital Statistics)

our calories in 1976, which is 50 percent more than the *12 percent* of the calories furnished to our grandparents in 1910.*

Imagine great-grandmother visiting her relatives in 1984. Today her breakfast might consist of donuts or sweet rolls and crunchy, heavily sugared cereal, colored in various hues. Her

---

*Reprinted from *Changing American Diet and Chemical Cuisine,* copyright 1980, which is available from the Center for Science in the Public Interest, 1501 16th Street N.W., Washington, DC 20036, for $4.00. Poster available for $3.95.

BLUEPRINT FOR HEALTH

orange juice could be made from water added to a heavily sweetened, artificially colored and flavored mix. Four or five cups of coffee mixed with sugar and a synthetic powder for cream would accompany her breakfast.

At lunch she would be fascinated to see our fast-food restaurants and the changing American diet. She would sample a milk shake or cola drink, French fries, and a greasy cheeseburger smothered with mayonnaise, mustard, catsup, onion, and pickle nestled in a lifeless bun. She might be aware of how many overweight people and poorly behaved children are also eating in the restaurant.

For dinner either she would be taken to a fancy restaurant or a fast-food fried-chicken place, or she would dine with the relatives.

The meal with the relatives might be preceded by cocktails, cheese and crackers, and dip and chips. Then comes the fat-marbled steak that dominates her plate. The potatoes would be instant mashed or a butter-and-sour-cream-smothered baked potato. Canned or frozen, heavily salted, overcooked vegetables might be served. The salad of iceberg lettuce and two tomato slices would be swimming in a sea of high-fat dressing. The soft white bread or rolls would stick to her dentures; she would rinse this off with her coffee or iced tea.

For dessert, there would be a choice of a hot-fudge sundae with chocolate-chip cookies, frozen pecan pie, or cake and frosting made from box mixes. Ice cream would be piled on the side and more coffee would be served.

After dinner great-grandmother complains of "heartburn."

With this kind of diet it is easy to see why the major killer diseases in our day are heart disease, stroke, arteriosclerosis, cancer, cirrhosis of the liver, and diabetes. Such diseases are caused by the body degenerating faster than it regenerates. And these diet-related diseases continue to grow more widespread.

Dr. Henry G. Beiler, who practiced medicine during the span of time we are considering, made an interesting statement in his book *Food Is Your Best Medicine,* published in 1963. He said, "When I first began to practice I would see two to three cases of cancer a year. Nowadays, I see six to eight a month."[8]

The Stanford Research Institute (San Jose, California) estimates that 80 percent of all cancer cases are caused by added artificial chemicals that humans encounter in their daily lives. Dr. Jacobson calls chemically adulterated food, "chemical cuisine," and warns us to beware of these foods. The following list is drawn from his scientific research.[9]

FOOD ADDITIVES—BEWARE

- Artificial Coloring—most are synthetic chemicals that do not occur in nature.
  - BHT (Butylated Hydroxytoluene)—antioxidant.
  - BVO (Brominated Vegetable Oil)—emulsifier.
  - Caffeine—stimulant.
  - Quinine—flavoring.
  - Saccharin—synthetic sweetener.
  - Salt—(Sodium Chloride)—flavoring.
  - Sodium Nitrite, Sodium Nitrate—preservative.
  - Sugar (Sucrose)—sweetener.
  - Artificial Flavoring.
  - BHA (Butylated Hydroxyanisole)—antioxidant.
  - MSG (Monosodium Glutamate)—flavor enhancer.
  - Polysorbate 60—emulsifier.
  - Sulfur Dioxide—Sodium Bisulfate—preservative, bleach.

Just for fun, use the "Food Additives—Beware" list to investigate your cupboards and refrigerator. Write down any foods containing those chemicals. Then remember—they could harm you.

_____

_____

_____

_____

_____

_____

_____

_____

_____

_____

_____

_____

But don't throw all these foods away. Simply use them up and replace them with unadulterated food.

Dr. George M. Briggs, chairman of the Nutritional Science Department at the University of California at Berkeley, observes, "The American public is eating a strange diet. We feed our farm animals better, giving them all the vitamins and minerals we take out of the food for humans."[10] I believe that if we refuse to become informed or blatantly choose to fill our bodies with foods we know are harmful, we could destroy ourselves.

Christians do not willfully inflict harm on their bodies, because, to a large degree, the condition of our bodies determines the effectiveness of our spiritual service. Christians must not ignore their physical health. Many avoid defiling their bodies with tobacco, alcohol, and harmful drugs, but they often ignore the defilement that comes through the nonnutritious foods they eat.[11]

God has said to the Christian, "Your body is a temple of the Holy Spirit who is in you, whom you have from God, and that you are not your own. For you have been bought with a price: therefore glorify God in your body" (1 Corinthians 6:19–20 NASB).

In chapter 1, I described my years of pain and suffering that were caused by my ignorance and disobedience in this area of my life. Out of love I beg you, brothers and sisters in Christ, to take heed so it won't happen to you.

When I encounter a problem, I always try to return to the fundamental facts. This can be applied in the area of nutrition. Basic foods, as close to their natural state as possible, are always the most nutritious. We should ask ourselves if the food we are about to devour is *junk* or *jewels*.

10 DO EATING PATTERNS REALLY MATTER? (AN APPLE A DAY KEEPS THE DOCTOR AWAY)

In the early part of the twentieth century, a dentist named Dr. Weston Price traveled all over the world seeking nutritional wisdom from primitive races. He found that dental caries, some physical deformities, physical and mental deterioration are directly related to poor diet.[1]

The following information is taken from Dr. Price's book *Nutrition and Physical Degeneration*. The book relates his studies of the eating habits and disease patterns among primitive cultures. One research program took place in the Torres Strait Islands north of Australia. As long as the native islanders lived without adopting the foods of modern civilization, they had nearly perfect bodies and an associated personality and character of high excellence. Dr. Price was impressed by the atmosphere of happiness, peace, and health radiating from their presence. Crime was practically nonexistent.

Dr. Price says, "In every tribal group regardless of age or location, there was sturdy development throughout their bodies, broad dental arches, and for all those who lived on their native foods, a close proximity to 100% immunity to dental cavity."[2]

Their diet consisted of seafood, dairy products, and fresh fruits and vegetables during the growing season. Nuts, seeds, and whole grains completed their diet. Most foods were eaten raw or very slightly cooked. Sweets were used only on special occasions.[3]

The Australian government later set up stores stocked with white flour, polished rice, canned goods, and sugar. The longer the primitive people were exposed to these foods, the more they suffered from physical degeneration. The first outward sign was loss of immunity to dental decay. Dr. Price stated, "In the succeeding generations studied there was a marked change in facial and dental arch form and a marked lowering of resistance to disease."[4]

In chapter 1 you found out my life was plagued with degenerative disease. Before these diseases struck, nearly every tooth in my mouth had been filled.

Write the names of each person who has had dental braces or bad teeth in your family.

_____

_____

_____

_____

Have they had any other health problems? List them.

_____

_____

_____

_____

Are their problems caused by infectious (pneumonia, tuberculosis) or degenerative diseases (cancer, heart, arthritis, asthma)?

Teeth and bones are made up of cells, as is the rest of the body. Take a look at the picture of a healthy human cell (Fig. 6.1). Man is assumed to be composed of approximately 600 trillion cells. As each second passes, some 50 million cells are formed to replace an equal number that have died in that time.[5]

The whole of the body consists of many types of cells. Can you name some?

_____

_____

_____

_____

_____

Look at your skin, nails, and hair and think of the cells making up these visible structures.

As you read and comprehend this sentence thank God for your healthy brain cells. Brain cells are necessary for our mind to function. Dr. Elie Shneour, a scientist and brain researcher, says in his book *The Malnourished Mind,* "At four years of age a child's brain has reached 90% of its adult weight. This rapid growth makes the brain particularly vulnerable to poor diet during pregnancy and the early years of life."[6]

Dr. Roger J. Williams, former director of the Clayton Foundation Biochemical Institute, explains, "Our brain cells ultimately get from blood only those nutrient elements that are furnished in the food we eat. What we eat therefore (or fail to eat) can directly affect how we feel, think, act, react and perceive the world around us."[7]

The body is the stage for a constant cellular nutritional melodrama. Body cells could be described as the heroine of this melodrama. These cells are working hard to function as a whole each minute of the day to produce a healthy body. In our melodrama we could describe the villains as the harmful nutritional thieves that rob our cells.

Our heroes are at work to protect us from the villains. The heroes are made up of the high quality, unadulterated, nutrient-filled foods we put into our bodies. To defeat the villains we must investigate to learn who they are.

Coffee, tea, alcohol, tobacco, sugar, salt (excessive), chemical food additives, and highly processed foods are unmasked as we open the investigation. Hiding in the wings are antibiotics, aspirin, diuretics, laxatives, birth control pills, and other drugs that also act like "nutritional thieves" or villains that rob the body of many nutrients.

An example is a diuretic drug prescribed for water retention (edema). Its use results in potassium and other minerals being kidnapped from the cells and lost in the urine. This upsets the cells' mineral balance. Nutrition plays a big role here. The heroes (orange juice, bananas, and hominy) increase the potassium intake and rescue the heroine from the threat of imbalance. But it isn't always possible to eat enough to correct the harmful effect of drugs.

Sugar is a stripped carbohydrate with only the empty calories remaining. Obesity can occur from overuse of this villainous nutritional thief. Sugar contains no vitamins, no minerals, no protein, no fat, and no fiber. Its overuse can cause one to incur a nutrient debt, even the bankruptcy of overnutrition (obesity) and malnutrition. Tooth decay is caused by consuming large quantities of sugar in candy, soft drinks, ice cream, cakes, and pies.

Breakfast starts the day. If you eat cereal, check the following list of cereals for sugar content. Note that Kellogg's Nutri-Grains are not listed. Devoid of sugar, they are nutritious heroes. Cooked cereals, oatmeal, whole-grain wheat, millet, grits, and brown rice possess greater nutrient value than the following.

THE SUGAR CONTENT OF READY-TO-EAT CEREALS

Product	Manufacturer	Total sugar (% dry weight)
Sugar Smacks	Kellogg	56.0
Apple Jacks	Kellogg	54.6
Fruit Loops	Kellogg	48.0
Sugar Corn Pops	Kellogg	46.0
Super Sugar Crisp	General Foods	46.0
Crazy Cow (chocolate)	General Mills	45.6
Corny Snaps	Kellogg	45.5
Frosted Rice Krinkles	General Foods	44.0
Frankenberry	General Mills	43.7
Cookie-Crisp, Vanilla	Ralston-Purina	43.5

Product	Manufacturer	Total sugar (% dry weight)
Cap'n Crunch's Crunch Berries	Quaker Oats	43.3
Cocoa Krispies	Kellogg	43.0
Cocoa Pebbles	General Foods	42.6
Fruity Pebbles	General Foods	42.5
Lucky Charms	General Mills	42.2
Cookie-Crisp, Chocolate	Ralston-Purina	41.0
Sugar Frosted Flakes	Kellogg	41.0
Quisp	Quaker Oats	40.7
Crazy Cow (strawberry)	General Mills	40.1
Cookie-Crisp, Oatmeal	Ralston-Purina	40.1
Cap'n Crunch	Quaker Oats	40.0
Count Chocula	General Mills	39.5
Alpha-Bits	General Foods	38.0
Honey Comb	General Foods	37.2
Frosted Rice	Kellogg	37.0
Trix	General Mills	35.9
Cocoa Puffs	General Mills	33.3
Cap'n Crunch, Peanut butter	Quaker Oats	32.2
Post Raisin Bran	General Foods	30.4
Golden Grahams	General Mills	30.0
Cracklin' Bran	Kellogg	29.0
Raisin Bran	Kellogg	29.0
C.W. Post, Raisin	General Foods	29.0
C. W. Post	General Foods	28.7
Frosted Mini-Wheats	Kellogg	26.0
Country Crisp	General Foods	22.0
Life, Cinnamon Flavor	Quaker Oats	21.0
100% Bran	Nabisco	21.0
All-Bran	Kellogg	19.0
Fortified Oat Flakes	General Foods	18.5
Life	Quaker Oats	16.0
Team	Nabisco	14.1
Grape-Nuts Flakes	General Foods	13.3
40% Bran Flakes	General Foods	13.0
Buc Wheat	General Mills	12.2
Product 19	Kellogg	9.9
Concentrate	Kellogg	9.3
Total	General Mills	8.3
Wheaties	General Mills	8.2
Rice Krispies	Kellogg	7.8
Grape-Nuts	General Foods	7.0
Special K	Kellogg	5.4

Product	Manufacturer	Total sugar (% dry weight)
Corn Flakes	Kellogg	5.3
Post Toasties	General Foods	5.0
Kix	General Mills	4.8
Rice Chex	Ralston-Purina	4.4
Corn Chex	Ralston-Purina	4.0
Wheat Chex	Ralston-Purina	3.5
Cheerios	General Mills	3.0
Shredded Wheat	Nabisco	0.6
Puffed Wheat	Quaker Oats	0.5
Puffed Rice	Quaker Oats	0.1

Source: Based on an analysis published in 1979 by the U.S. Department of Agriculture of cereals that account for 90 percent of those purchased by Americans.

Note: For a more reasonable balance of nutrients, concentrate on those cereals that contain less than 10 percent sugar. Note that most of these are the brands you grew up with, in contrast to the sugar-laden brands introduced during recent decades. If additional sweetening is desired, garnish your cereal with fresh fruit.

Are there any "nutritional thieves" in your life? What are they?

_____

_____

_____

_____

_____

What better substitutes could you use?

Drugs are sometimes a necessity and should always be used as prescribed by your physician. If you take prescription drugs daily, it is possible that you may need more of the B-complex vitamins (especially B6, B12, and niacin), vitamin C, vitamin E, and potassium to counteract the depletion caused by many prescription drugs.

The heroes trying to save our cells deserve more attention. Hero menus follow. You might want to try some of them. The menu suggestions will cover three meals a day. The first is breakfast, which derives its name from "breaking the fast." This meal makes or breaks the day. It has been proven that skipping breakfast over the years accelerates the aging process.

Dinner menus will be given for the noontime meal. These meals will be larger than the evening or supper meals. Although this is the ideal way to eat, it is not always possible. Heavier meals should be consumed before one expends the most energy.

Snacks will be included to help those who have blood sugar problems or are constantly in a state of fatigue. Remember when you eat snacks, six very small meals would be best. Watch your calorie intake so you won't gain weight. Remember, each person is unique and these are only basic menus.

EATING-ADVENTURE MENUS

As you eat the following foods, note any problems under comments. You may find foods you are allergic to.

Day 1

Breakfast

Oatmeal cooked with raisins and cinnamon
Yogurt with fresh fruit

Morning Snack

Citrus fruit

Dinner

Oven-fried caraway chicken
Apple salad
Green peas with mint
Pears with ricotta cheese

Afternoon Snack

Bread or Crackers

Supper

Open face turkey sandwich on rye bread
with tomato and sprouts
Tossed salad
Fresh fruit

Comments: _____

_____

Day 2

Breakfast

Orange slices or juice
Poached eggs—one large or two medium
Whole-grain toast

Morning Snack

Yogurt

Dinner

Baked turbot
Parsley buttered noodles
Garlic green beans

Afternoon Snack

Pear

Supper

Lavosh covered with steamed vegetables
(carrots, celery, zucchini, onion,
green pepper) and cheese
Baked apple

Comments: _____

_____

Day 3

Breakfast

Whole-grain pancakes covered with
yogurt or cottage cheese
Fresh fruit or applesauce and nuts

Morning Snack

Fresh peach

Dinner

Roast turkey
Brown rice amandine
Broccoli with caraway sauce
Tossed green salad

Afternoon Snack

Celery stuffed with peanut butter

Supper

Cottage cheese or yogurt with
Pineapple, pear, peach, and banana chunks

Zucchini bread

Comments: _____

_____

Day 4

Breakfast

Homemade granola with banana slices
Turkey sausage

Morning Snack

Toast or crackers

Dinner

Chicken parmesan
Spinach souffle
Baked potato with parsley
Tomato salad
Spiced prunes

Afternoon Snack

Apple

Supper

Chicken vegetable soup
Tossed romaine salad with vegetables

Whole-grain crackers

Comments: _____

_____

Day 5

Breakfast

Grapefruit
Hot apple granola
Corn muffins

Morning Snack

Peach

Dinner

Sirloin casserole
Baked sweet potato
Zucchini—steamed with tomatoes
Fresh fruit compote

Afternoon Snack

Yogurt

Supper

Navy bean soup
Corn muffins
Steamed carrots with almonds and dill

Comments: _____

_____

Day 6

Breakfast

Scrambled eggs with low-fat cheese and tomato slices
Bran muffins

Morning Snack

Fresh fruit

Dinner

New England pot roast with potatoes, carrots,
celery, and onions
Tossed salad with vegetables and beets

Afternoon Snack

Bran muffin

Supper

Lentil soup
Tossed salad
Corn bread

Comments: _____

_____

Day 7

Breakfast

Cooked cracked wheat with sliced peaches and banana
Toasted whole-grain English muffin
Peach

Morning Snack

Whole-wheat bagel

Dinner

Lemon-broiled salmon steak
Rice with peas and green beans
Carrot salad with raisins

Melon and fresh fruit

Afternoon Snack

Apple

Supper

Split pea soup
Corn muffin
Tossed salad

Comments: _____

_____

One of my patients told me he was a meat-and-potatoes man. He said, "I don't like anything else." As we looked over his past health problems, he finally admitted he needed help and agreed to try some new foods.

Variety is the spice of life. The broader the base of foods we eat, the greater the insurance against missing some of the vitamins, minerals, enzymes, and amino acids.

Look back over the "Eating-Adventure Menu" and make out some menus of your own. Incorporate the knowledge you have gained from the study of this book.

MY SELF-DESIGNED EATING ADVENTURE MEALS
Day 1

Breakfast

_____

_____

_____

Morning Snack

_____

Dinner

_____

_____

_____

_____

Afternoon Snack

_____

Supper

_____

_____

_____

Comments: _____

_____

Day 2

Breakfast

_____

_____

_____

Morning Snack

_____

Dinner

_____

_____

_____

_____

Afternoon Snack

_____

Supper

_____

_____

Comments: _____

_____

Twenty years ago when I was wracked with the pain of arthritis and depressed about my failing health, a wise friend suggested I change my diet. After listening half-heartedly to her suggestions, I thought of every objection I could. My quick retort was, "But it takes too much time. I'm too busy." She tried to help me, but I wasn't interested. I forgot to take into account the wasted hours spent in bed while I was sick. Proverbs 1:5 states, "A wise man will hear and increase in learning, And a man of understanding will acquire wise counsel" (NASB). I was neither hearing nor increasing my learning, and I did not want wise counsel.

As my health continued to disintegrate, I finally faced the fact that I had to do something: I had to learn how to change my basic eating habits. I began to realize that if I took a little time now, maybe I could save a lot of time and misery in the future. I have discovered some time-saving tips that I try to follow.

To save valuable time and be prepared, stock up on staple foods. Here is a list of essentials in my kitchen:

Oatmeal, oat bran, wheat bran, muesli, corn grits, millet, rice cereal, wheat flakes

Whole wheat and buckwheat flour, corn meal, brown rice, wheat germ, brewers yeast, nonfat dry milk

Dry beans, split peas, lentils, potatoes, onions, carrots, apples, citrus fruits

Whole grain crackers and breads, pita bread, tortillas, cereal snack-mix, unsalted corn chips, graham crackers, rice cakes

Whole wheat lasagna and spaghetti, spinach noodles, artichoke macaroni

Raisins, prunes, dried apricots

Mexican salsa, eggs, pickles

Sesame and sunflower seeds, almonds, pecans, nut butters (sesame, almond, peanut), and sprouting seeds

Low-fat string cheese, baby swiss, hoop and low-fat cottage cheese and yogurt

Herbs and herb teas (camomile, peppermint, lemon mist, orange spice, apple)

Spices and vegetable seasonings to replace salt, such as Mrs. Dash,® Vegit,® Spike,® Jensen's Broth®

These ingredients can be stored in attractive covered glass jars and used as counter decorations. Grains, nuts, seeds, cereals, and cheeses should be refrigerated.

My freezer contains juices, corn on the cob, peas, broccoli, cauliflower, strawberries, peaches, blueberries, and applesauce. These were purchased in season and frozen. Tasty home-cooked meals are also frozen ready for company and busy days. Frozen chickens, turkey breast, cornish hens, stew beef and roasts make meal planning fun instead of drudgery.

Meal preparation is hurried along by chopping vegetables in a food processor. A pressure cooker or microwave oven saves cooking time. The crockpot meal begins in the morning and is ready for dinner.

Salad greens are washed, and a salad spinner dries them. Refrigerate them in a large covered plastic bowl. A blender makes instant soups, spreads, sauces, and shakes and grates cheese and chops nuts. Cook vegetables held in a steamer basket over one inch of water in a pot. This is quick and conserves nutrients.

Fasten plastic bags with clip clothespins for speed in opening and closing.

Don't forget to make out weekly menus and grocery lists. Cook several meals at once to make maximum use of time.

If you are going to convince yourself to shape up your diet, you must be convinced it is worthwhile.

Collin H. Dong, M.D., in his book *New Hope for the Arthritic,* reminds the reader of the importance of diet in disease. If diet will help overcome chronic degenerative disease, think what it will do to keep a healthy body from deteriorating.

In 1931 Dr. Dong graduated from Stanford Medical School and interned at San Francisco General Hospital. Seven years later at the age of thirty-five he was afflicted by arthritis. As the crippling pain in his joints worsened, he developed a severe generalized skin rash. For three years he lived on large doses of aspirin—the only medically prescribed treatment. Common side effects from heavy aspirin usage include stomach ulcers and ringing in the ears.

"I had given very little thought or consideration to the problem of food and its effect on the human body," Dr. Dong states, "except that I knew I had to eat to live and work. In medical school I had *no training in the science of nutrition.*"

One day Dr. Dong remembered what his father had said to all nine of his children when any of them became ill. Translated from Chinese into English his advice was, "Sickness enters through the mouth, and catastrophe comes out of the mouth."

Like many people who are steeped in technology, higher education, and scientific knowledge, Dr. Dong had forgotten the simple way in which he was raised.

His diet for his first two decades was a simple Chinese diet, consisting mainly of beef, chicken, fish, vegetables, and rice— never desserts. He explains, "At age twenty-eight when I started to practice medicine, I gradually changed to a diet like that of most Americans. My usual breakfast was orange or tomato juice, ham or bacon with eggs, coffee with sugar and cream; for lunch, it would be such things as canned soups, roast beef, hot breads, sandwiches, apple pie à la mode, all washed down with a soft drink; for dinner, I usually ate out at restaurants in the city." He goes on, "In fact I was eating like a pig."

Seven years later the result of this dietary change was a weight gain of forty pounds and a wheelchair to carry his arthritic body.

Dr. Dong relates his experiment: "I went back to the Chinese 'poor-man's diet' that I had been brought up on. I finally settled on seafood, vegetables, and rice as the best diet for me. . . . To my utter amazement in a few short weeks there was a metamorphosis. I was able to shave again for my skin had become soft and pliable and did not weep. I was agile again, for I went from 195 pounds to 150 pounds, which is the weight I maintain today. I was able to play golf again, for the pain and stiffness in my joints disappeared. I had almost complete remission of my crippling disease."

Dr. Dong is now in his seventies, and the last I heard he is still practicing medicine every day and playing golf every Wednesday afternoon. His arthritis is a disease of the past.[8]

A close personal friend of mine went to Dr. Dong when she developed crippling arthritis. Thanks to him, her diet was changed, and she too is free of pain and disability. She is even able to enjoy playing tennis again.

The words of wisdom Dr. Dong has imparted to the thousands of patients he has successfully treated for rheumatic disease include:

Nutrition is related to health and illness.
Hazards of eating include:
    Processed foods
    Artificial flavorings
    Artificial colorings
    Chemical preservatives
    Other additives
    Eating foods to which you are allergic[9]

The late Dr. Ben Feingold, who worked with hyperactive children, found by eliminating these same foods in children's diets, their behavior often improved, and school performance was upgraded.

Do eating patterns really matter? What are your thoughts?
While you make your list, eat "an apple today to keep the doctor away."

_____

_____

_____

_____

11 ARE THERE ANY PROBLEMS BESIDES FOOD THAT CAUSE ILLNESS?

MENTAL ATTITUDE

David Messenger, M.D., believes bad feelings produce bad body chemistry. He has shown that anger, bitterness, and hatred can raise blood pressure and cause ulcers, colitis, rashes, headaches, and heart attacks. Constant negative emotions deplete the adrenal glands, the shock absorbers of the body, and cause *dis*-ease. In addition, his research has shown that positive attitudes produce self-confidence, joy, happiness, peace of mind, and create a sense of *ease* within the body.[1]

This should not surprise us. Long before the time of Christ, Solomon wrote: "Anxiety in the heart of man weighs it down" (Proverbs 12:25 NASB).

Dr. Albert Schweitzer realized the importance of humor as therapy for his tired hospital staff at Lambarene. Schweitzer always had a humorous story or two to tell at the dinner table. The laughter seemed to rejuvenate the exhausted young doctors and nurses.[2]

In his book *Anatomy of an Illness*, Norman Cousins tells how laughing at "Candid Camera" and old Marx Brothers' films controlled his pain for nearly two hours at a time.[3] At the time, he had ankylosing spondylitis, which meant the connective tissue in his spine was disintegrating. The blood sedimentation rate in this disease elevates. His was dangerously high. Blood was drawn before and after he laughed at the funny movies. His sedimentation would drop and stay down after each episode.[4]

On a scale of one to ten, rate your mental attitude. Circle where you fall.

Negative Attitudes   Positive Attitudes

1   2   3   4   5   6   7   8   9   10

Do you have a good sense of humor? _____.

Start spending time with friends who make you laugh. Insert their names here:

_____

_____

Call them up and plan to get together.

SMOKING

The B-complex vitamins and vitamin C are depleted by smoking. Smoking causes cancer, emphysema, heart disease, and other chronic diseases. A government publication identifies cigarette smoking as the single most important preventable cause of death.

Even though these facts are known, people often say, "I have to die of something." That is true, but the torture and painful lingering death associated with these diseases should be considered. Lung cancer usually spreads cancer cells to other parts of the body so that people may die of brain or liver cancer because of smoking.

When I was stricken with tuberculosis, my lung doctor was considered one of the best in the Midwest. On my first visit to his office, after my hospital release, I was stunned to see the ashtray on his desk full of cigarette butts. As he puffed away he said to me, "Now, I don't want you to ever smoke. Do you smoke now?" I peered into his eyes, set my jaw, and replied, "No, I don't smoke, and you shouldn't fill my lungs with your smoke." He ignored my plea because he wasn't ready to make that commitment. As we got to know him better my husband and I tried to get him to stop smoking. When we saw him two years ago, we were relieved to hear he had finally quit.

DRINKING

Alcohol depletes vitamin A, B complex, potassium, and other nutrients. The Surgeon General's report, *Healthy People,* connects the consumption of large amounts of alcohol with cancer of the larynx, esophagus, oral cavity, and liver. It isn't proven whether the cause relates to the nutritional deficiencies occurring from heavy drinking or contaminants from the manufacturing of alcohol.[5]

In 1979 there were 10 million problem drinkers in America. More than 30,000 Americans died from cirrhosis of the liver in 1977. Alcohol is an indirect cause of many of the 150,000 deaths annually from accidents, homicides, and suicides.[6]

SLEEP AND RELAXATION

The proper amount of sleep is essential for abundant energy. Authorities agree that a minimum amount of sleep for most people is seven hours. If your demands are higher and you ignore them, you may suffer the consequences. During rest and sleep your mind and body recharge themselves.

Charles T. Kuntzleman, Ed.D., in his book *Maximum Personal Energy*, feels sleep is essential to give the body rest from the constant bombardment of stimuli experienced daily. Revitalization occurs during sleep when the nervous system is no longer being stimulated.[7]

Researchers feel that it is difficult to make up for lost sleep. Some believe that each time you fail to get an adequate amount of sleep you lose extra brain cells; cells that cannot be replaced.[8]

If you go for two days without sleep you will lose your ability to concentrate. Three days without sleep will cause difficulty thinking, seeing and hearing, and you may have hallucinations.

Six years ago a young man set a goal to beat the Guinness world record for the most consecutive hours of playing tennis. He chose a tennis club near our home. We went each day to watch him play. Later in an interview he told me, "Between seventy-nine to eighty hours I lost all sense of reality and thought I was dreaming. . . . Even only after eighteen hours I was depressed, had mental fatigue, and couldn't concentrate." He stopped only long enough to take food, rest a short time, and have his vital signs monitored. The third day while we watched him play, his helpers had to force him onto the court, show him how to hit the ball, and quiet his rebellious yelling. He was confused, had a wild look in his eyes, and was belligerent. He beat the record only to have it surpassed in two weeks. In retrospect he mused, "I would never go out in public drunk, but my behavior was just as offensive." His body suffered from the continuous bombardment of stimulation to his nervous system accompanied by no sleep.

How much sleep do you get each night? _____. Is this enough? _____.

If you suffer from insomnia, it could be caused by a nutritional deficiency according to biochemist Roger Williams, Ph.D. The following guidelines to overcome insomnia are found in Charles T. Kuntzleman's book *Maximum Personal Energy:*

1. Do not eat a heavy meal before going to bed.
2. Do not watch TV or read an exciting book before retiring.
3. Take a warm bath before retiring.
4. Drink a warm beverage just before bed.
5. Occupy yourself with a quiet hobby.
6. Take a leisurely walk before retiring.
7. Consciously try to relax the muscles of your body. Start with your feet and work your way up your body.
8. Try reading a very boring or dull book.
9. Get involved in a good overall aerobic fitness program.[9]

If you try these suggestions and still have insomnia you might try taking calcium and magnesium at bedtime or tryptophan (an amino acid). A glass of milk or a cup of warm camomile tea may also be beneficial.

EXERCISE, FRESH AIR, AND SUNSHINE

The late Paul Dudley White, dean of American cardiologists, declared, "The brain needs to be well fed with oxygen and other chemicals, and its waste products need to be removed. Only the blood can do that. For its optimal function, therefore, the brain must have a good fresh supply of blood which is delivered by a good heart and good blood vessels which should be kept in good condition."[10]

Often, when I have suggested exercise as a part of the program for my counselees, they list their excuses. Some would say, "I will follow the diet, drink the water, get more rest, and take the vitamins and mineral supplements, but I hate to exercise." The counselees most interested in exercise had previously suffered major illnesses often related to the cardiovascular system. They realized the necessity for exercise and were sorry they hadn't started sooner.

Dr. Kenneth Cooper's prescription for better health and more stamina is what he calls *aerobic* exercise. Aerobic means "with oxygen."[11] Driving to work, sitting at a desk, watching TV, and being a spectator at sports events are *not* aerobic exercises. Dr. Cooper lists running, swimming, cycling, walking, running in place, handball, basketball, and squash as the best aerobic exercises.[12] I would add aerobic dance, jumping rope, and jogging on a trampoline (rebounding).

Almost everyone can exercise by walking. We can continue to walk as we get older, even if we become limited in other ways. I suggest you start slowly and build up to two miles in thirty minutes daily. Walking in the fresh air and sunshine will enable your mind to relax as you view the beauty of nature.

STRESS

A run-away truck rolled into a woman pedestrian as she walked next to a brick building. She braced her back and legs against the building and stopped the truck with her outstretched arms and hands to keep from being crushed. After the truck was removed she collapsed and had to be treated medically. Although she had received bruises, no bones were broken, for her supernatural strength had been generated by stress.

Do you have stress in your life? Life is full of hassles and day-to-day stresses. Stress by itself can be either beneficial or harmful. A person's attitude toward stress and how it is handled makes the difference.

What kinds of recurring stress are hardest for you to handle?

_____

_____

_____

What are you most frustrated about?

_____

_____

_____

The two ways to cope with stress are to either change the negative attitude to a positive one or get rid of the stressor. When people elect to change their attitudes, they jump into the driver's seat and make stress work for them. It can no longer pressure them.

Dr. Hans Selye, world famous authority on stress, wrote a book entitled *Stress Without Distress*. In it he says, "Try to keep your mind constantly on the pleasant aspects of life and on actions which can improve your situation. Try to forget everything that is irrevocably ugly or painful. This is perhaps the most efficient way of minimizing stress by what I have called voluntary mental diversion."

Dr. Selye, believes that when we perceive stress distressfully, it can cause real physical changes in our bodies. The end result of this situation makes the body more vulnerable to the rapid effects of aging.[13] And degenerative disease is related to the aging process.

The Bible suggests excellent ways to keep stress from becoming distress. Philippians 4:8–9 commands: "Finally, brethren, whatever is true, whatever is honorable, whatever is right, whatever is pure, whatever is lovely, whatever is of good repute, if there is any excellence and if anything worthy of praise, let your mind dwell on these things" (NASB).

Ephesians 4:31–32 states: "Let all bitterness and wrath and

anger and clamor and slander be put away from you, along with all malice. And be kind to one another, tender hearted, forgiving each other, just as God in Christ also has forgiven you" (NASB).

Corrie Ten Boom encountered the stress of persecution at the hands of the Nazis while imprisoned in one of their death camps. She took hold of her stress by repeating often, "However deep the pit, God's love is deeper still."

If believers follow God's instructions, they can gain inner peace and master the circumstances, and they won't be victimized by stress.

DRUGS

Although millions of lives have been saved by drugs, there is an epidemic of iatrogenic disorders that are often caused by some physicians' treatment prescribed for their patients. Many people have told me their health was rapidly disintegrating so they changed doctors. The new doctor found out that the combination of previously prescribed drugs was the root cause of their problem.

Drugs are toxic to some extent and produce dietary deficiencies by destroying nutrients. They either use the nutrients up, prevent their absorption, increase their excretion, or chemically take their place. Most people are ill before they take drugs, and the body's nutrients are already somewhat depleted. Extremely deficient people will have more damage from drug toxicity. Drugs taken over a long period of time can be especially harmful.

When taking drugs, you should concentrate on eating highly nutritious meals to prevent trouble. Protein foods and green leafy vegetables are essential.

Liver damage, digestive problems, allergies, stomach ulcers, diabetes, and colitis have all been related to drug toxicity.

Drugs cause stress and therefore increase the need for vitamin C, pantothenic acid, B-complex vitamins, and vitamin E. Some drugs cause mineral depletion of zinc, calcium, magnesium, potassium, and other minerals.

AIR AND WATER POLLUTION

When we moved to Phoenix in 1967, the air-pollution level was low. At that time trace amounts of carbon monoxide, sulfur dioxide, oxides of nitrogen, ozone, hydrogen sulfide, and methane were present in the air. Even the purest air has some contaminants in small amounts. It is only when the pollutants are present at a high level that air pollution threatens the human being.

Over the past seventeen years the air quality in Phoenix has deteriorated. Now frequent alerts are broadcast in the newspaper and on radio and television, warning people with respiratory ailments to stay indoors. It is an understatement to say that air pollution in many of the major cities has become a health hazard. Toxic minerals such as lead find their way into plants and then into animals or humans that eat the plants.

Many foreign substances present in the body at high levels can threaten health. These substances reach our bodies through the air we breathe and the water we drink.

It is obvious that a problem exists. A problem that affects everyone, but it could possibly be offset by a nutritious diet.

This past week I received three disturbing phone calls. The first was from a twenty-eight-year-old female who suffered from cancer (malignant melanoma) of the eye three years ago. She told me, "My cancer has returned and is now in my spine and liver." I wanted to cry; she is so young. I thought, *If she had been started on a nutritious diet and supplements as a child, I wonder if it would have helped.*

The second phone call was from a family friend I had watched grow from a child to a young lady. She is married and the mother of two small daughters. She calmly said, "I am three months pregnant, and last week the doctor found a malignant lump in my breast." She continued, "Tomorrow they are removing my breast and checking the lymph nodes." Then she said, "I want to get on a good nutrition program." I reflected that if she had started on this program as a child, it might have made a difference.

The third phone call was from the sister of a forty-four-year-old man. Three years ago her brother had the lymph glands removed from his neck. Hodgkin's disease was diagnosed. Now the cancer has started to metastasize. He is desperate for help. Once again, I am reminded of the questions: Would things have been different if he had started caring for his nutritional needs as a youngster? Why is cancer attacking so many young people?

My challenge to you as you read these last pages is to seriously think about your health, your children's health, and even the health of the unborn babies. Make an effort to "do something" to help lessen health catastrophies.

Health, like freedom, is most appreciated after it is lost.

What can a person do to protect himself against these pollutants? Concentrate on eating the most nutritious diet possible. Eat foods like grains, nuts, eggs, milk, cheese, and dried beans, which contain sulfur-bearing amino acids. Apples, bananas, carrots and the white of the citrus peel are high in pectin. All these foods help prevent the build up of toxic materials. The following dietary supplements may give added protection: Vitamins A, C, and E, which help protect the body's tissues against harmful pollutants.

POOR BOWEL HABITS

Executive Health Newsletter reported that in 1980 Americans spent 200 million dollars buying 800 different laxatives. These figures indicate that many people are concerned about their bowel habits.[14]

Regular use of purging-type laxatives is addictive and depletes the body of nutrients. When bowel function has been poor for a long time, a person needs to take definite steps toward improving the situation. Neither constipation nor diarrhea are normal conditions; both conditions should act as red flags to alert the individual. Measures should be taken to normalize the function.

It is often necessary to do a colon cleansing regime to start on an improved elimination program. This can include taking one teaspoon of a bulk producing intestinal cleanser (such as powdered psyllium seed) plus one tablespoon of liquid bentonite in juice and two herbal laxative tablets at bedtime. Drink one full eight-ounce glass of water before retiring. The next morning repeat all but the herbal laxative before breakfast. Repeat this only when necessary later.

The next steps in the program would be to drink your personal water allowance daily (see chapter 4), and add more fiber to your diet by eating raw fruits, vegetables, whole grains, and legumes. Alfalfa tablets can provide bulk too. Oat and wheat bran are high in fiber and can be added to the diet.

Yogurt, keifer, and acidophilus milk promote the growth of good bacteria in the intestines. For this reason, when you have taken massive doses of antibiotics, which kill all bacteria good and bad, ingestion of one of these is imperative to prevent debilitating diarrhea. Prunes, figs, and fresh pears contain fiber and have a laxative effect for some people.

Exercise is another boost in overcoming bowel problems.

Reread this chapter and list the habits you have decided to change.

_____

_____

_____

_____

_____

How do people get started changing bad habits? It is self-defeating to say, "I have to quit doing this or that." It is better and more productive to affirm positively, "I will do this instead of that." A person needs to focus on a positive substitution for a negative habit.

For instance, worry is a negative habit. It is impossible to worry and pray at the same time. When a person begins to worry, he needs to stop and praise God for the good things that he does have. He should claim God's promises to care for him and remember His never-ending love.

As you decide your plan of attack against bad habits list what positive substitutes you will use.

Bad Habit   Positive Substitution

_____   _____

_____   _____

_____   _____

_____   _____

_____   _____

_____   _____

12 MOST COMMONLY ASKED QUESTIONS (HOW CAN I KNOW WHAT'S RIGHT FOR ME?)

Each time I have had a speaking engagement over the last two years, I ask the audience to list their unanswered questions on a sheet of paper. On the following pages I will answer some of the most commonly asked questions. Although these answers come from my knowledge and experience in the health field, this information should *not* be misinterpreted as diagnosis or prescription; the information is for educational purposes only. For specific problems you should consult your physician and abide by his decision for diagnosis, prescription, and treatment.

Since each person is biochemically unique, there are no pat answers to any single problem. You must become aware of your own body and how it reacts. All illness comes from a breakdown of the body's immune defense system, which can be caused by nutrient deficiencies from either poor food, poor absorption by the body, or depletion from stress or other factors. The following suggestions will be general, and my primary focus will be on building the body's immune system so that it can do the work of protecting itself.

ATTITUDES

Q. Does a proper diet help marital and family relationships?

A. Relationships are dependent upon many variables. Spiritual and emotional maturity affect relationships more than anything.

Everyone is aware of the way stress, lack of sleep, and illness affect one's outlook on life. Many scientists and some medical doctors are beginning to believe that by restoring nutritional balance in the body, the mind and emotional health will improve. Yes, a proper diet can affect marital and family relationships for the better.

Also, if vitamins and minerals are not supplied in the necessary amounts, the immune system will weaken and the body, mind, and emotions will suffer. *Warning:* Do not rush out and purchase these vitamin and mineral supplements in large doses. Correct your eating habits and watch for positive improvement. Then you may want to add a balanced multiple *vitamin-mineral* supplement, plus extra vitamin C, E, and B complex. Some people need extra calcium and magnesium.

ANTI-AGING

Q. What can we do about the aging process?

A. Eat a nutritionally balanced diet that is especially rich in vegetables, grains, and fruits. Be sure to get enough protein. Work on having a positive mental attitude. Keep busy and challenged. Exercise the body and supply the necessary vitamins and minerals. Add a good vitamin-mineral supplement, B-complex vitamins; take vitamins C, E, and A. As they grow older many people need additional minerals: calcium, magnesium (preferably together), and zinc (preferably with vitamin A). Current research is inconclusive regarding dosages of selenium and chromium as age retardants.

ADDITIVES

Q. What about the additives and preservatives in soft drinks?

A. They are injurious! The phosphorous destroys calcium in the body. The artificial sweeteners and other chemicals have not proved safe and some are carcinogens. Sugar rots your teeth and abuses the body. The caffeine that is found in some soft drinks is a detrimental heart-stimulating drug.

Q. Is MSG (monosodium glutamate) harmful?

A. Yes, if you are allergic to it, and many people are. Asthma attacks, nausea, and headaches are all symptoms associated with intake of MSG. The so-called Chinese Restaurant Syndrome happens when people highly allergic to MSG eat heavy doses of it in Chinese food. Such people suddenly become ill.

Q. Is commercially made ice cream full of chemicals?

A. There are more than sixty chemical additives that *might* be added to your ice cream. Check the labels. You may find artificial flavorings instead of real fruit flavor. Carrageenan, gum tragabanth, carbohymethylcellulose, polysorbate 65 or 80, sodium hexametaphosphate are only a few chemicals used. Commercial ice-cream laws are deficient in that they do not require proper listing of ingredients.

Q. What do manufactured chemicals do to the body?

A. The science community does not know what many of the chemical food additives and preservatives do to the human body. Research has proven some of them cause cancer, intestinal lesions, heart damage, and organ and kidney damage in animals. Many have been removed from the market and many others probably should be.

ALLERGIES

Q. What are some of the most common allergens?

A. Many of the three thousand chemicals used in processed foods may be common allergens. Allergists tell us that the number of allergic people is increasing geometrically annually. Many people are allergic to some very common foods: chocolate, wheat, oranges, milk, sugar, corn, and eggs. Dust, animal hair, and commercial chemicals are common environmental allergens.

If you suffer from allergies, you need to do a health review, improve your diet, eliminate stress, exercise each day, and take extra food supplements to strengthen your weakened immune system. Dr. Arthur Coco's book *The Pulse Test* may be helpful in identifying some of your allergens. He believes food allergens elevate the pulse rate after consumption.[1]

ALCOHOLISM

Q. Is alcoholism a disease? Can improved nutrition help?

A. Dr. Roger J. Williams believes alcoholism is a physical disease and that it is usually curable. He recognizes psychiatry, medicine, religion, and nutrition as important facets of rehabilitation. An alcoholic should eat high-quality protein, fresh vegetables and fruits, and whole grains. Refined foods, including sugar and syrups should be avoided.[2] Dr. Williams recommends adding a good food supplement containing B complex, A, C, and E vitamins plus a multiple mineral tablet.[3] His research has also shown the amino acid L glutamine might be helpful.[4]

DEGENERATIVE DISEASE

Q. What is the best way to care for asthma, arthritis, diabetes, hypoglycemia, cancer, high blood pressure, heart problems, and depression?

A. All these are diseases that need to be supervised by a medical doctor. Nutrition isn't a cure-all. God did, however, design the human body and the food that keeps it healthy. One side of the coin shows how eating junk foods and ignoring good eating habits spells trouble. The other side of the coin shows that eating highly nutritious food, as suggested in this book, will strengthen the body's cells toward good health. Healthy cells can fight the battle of disease better. It is logical to assume that when a person is fortified by good nutrition health may improve.

The following letter is from a woman who attended one of my nutrition lectures: "I have had rheumatoid arthritis for fourteen years. My hands have been operated on thirty times and my left leg seven times. All the research drugs I took never stopped the progress of my disease. My prayers were answered when I was led to a holistic doctor, who changed my diet and started me taking food supplements. I am no longer losing my joints. My life was spent in bed before, and now I am able to be active."

Q. What is *Chelation Therapy,* and when should it be given?
A. Chelation therapy is a controversial treatment used for hardening of the arteries, diabetic gangrene, stroke damage, senility, and eye problems. An intravenous solution containing the chemical EDTA is infused into the arteries. EDTA is a

chemical channel blocker and helps pull calcium from atherosclerotic plaque and other areas of the body where it deposits such as tendons, joints, and ligaments. It doesn't seem to remove calcium from bones or teeth.

In *The Chelation Answer,* Morton Walker, D.P.N., and Garry Gordon, M.D., say, "Diagnostic tests taken before and after chelation therapy reveal that areas of impaired circulation are often restored to normal." They believe blood can circulate better after the clogging material is removed from the arterial wall.[5]

Q. Can anything be done to prevent cancer?

A. I average at least two telephone calls a month from people who have cancer. Invariably when I ask if they have eaten a nutritious diet in the past, the answer is no. When asked if they have taken food supplements, the answer is usually no. If one is eating dangerously, negative consequences result. Cancer strikes when the immune system is weak and the body is sick.

It is necessary to think and plan ahead. By choosing food carefully, exercising, resting the body, practicing a positive mental attitude, and taking extra nourishment through food supplements, one is at least trying to stay healthy. The difficulty is in getting well after being sick. The easiest approach is staying well.

Q. Is cancer related to the herpes virus?

A. Research is currently being done on this subject. A few reports state that some types of cancer may be related, but proof is not yet available. One researcher is using an amino acid lysine to treat herpes and suggesting it as a possible preventative of some forms of cancer.

Q. Can diet help diverticulosis?

A. Diverticulosis is a fingerlike projection coming off the colon. The modern highly refined low-residue diet is responsible for this condition. Current research shows that including more soluble and insoluble fiber in the diet will help eliminate this problem. Fresh vegetables, fruits, whole-grain breads, and cereals are all good high-fiber foods.

EXERCISE

Q. If we do strenuous exercise do we need more protein?

A. Research shows the daily requirement of protein for men, women, and children is adequate for even strenuous exercise. Body building of muscle tissue is the exception to the rule. More protein is required to build the muscle mass. Weight lifters should add extra protein.

Q. Does exercise give more energy and stamina? What kind of exercise could arthritics do?

A. Aerobic exercise oxygenates the blood better, moves the nutrients faster, and removes the toxins quicker. An ultimate result of such exercise is increased stamina and energy. If exercise makes you tired, reevaluate the type of exercise and the time of day you do it. If you are exhausted when you start exercising, it may stress your glandular and organ system and cause fatigue. Arthritics can exercise best when immersed in water. Some can exercise on a mini-trampoline more easily. Fast walking is good exercise for arthritics.

FOOD

Q. Do we eat too much red meat, eggs, and cheese?

A. Some cardiovascular physicians would say yes. Elevated cholesterol and triglyceride counts are warning signals. The high rate of heart disease in this country is alarming. Some researchers believe a high-fat diet may be one contributing factor in heart disease. Therefore, they think it may be safer to cut down on the amount of high-fat red meats, dairy products, and cholesterol present in egg yolks. But the medical community is not in total agreement.

Q. What can we eat when dining out?

A. Most restaurants serve baked or broiled fish, chicken, and lean meat. Baked potato, rice, vegetables, and rye bread are usually available. Soups and salads are generally on the menu too. Just skip the sour cream, butter, gravies, sauces, coffee, and desserts. Nevertheless, no matter what you order, you are likely to get too much salt in restaurant food.

Q. Are brown sugar and honey good replacements for sugar?
A. These are simple carbohydrates like sugar and involve the pancreas in like manner. Unprocessed raw honey may be a little more nutritious, but any of these sweeteners should be used sparingly.

Q. When at club meetings or church functions how can I avoid desserts, coffee, cakes, and cookies?
A. Either abstain or take a fruit plate or vegetable tray with dip to share. I have found that when I serve these things with a dessert too, the fruit and vegetables are the first to go. One needs to encourage others to serve healthy food by example.

Q. What are the best foods for a child's diet?
A. The same foods that are best for adults. If your children rebel at your diet changes, I would suggest you read *How to Convert the Kids From What They Eat to What They Oughta* by Polly Greenberg.[6] You can't beat fruits and vegetables, beans, whole-grain breads and cereals, milk, small amounts of fish, chicken, eggs, and low-fat cheeses.

Q. What seasonings are available in place of salt?
A. Vegit, Spike, Jensen's Broth, and Mrs. Dash are all healthy, tasty seasonings. Herbs can also flavor food: allspice, bay leaf, basil, caraway, cayenne pepper, cinnamon, celery, cloves, cumin, dill, garlic, ginger, horseradish, onion, oregano, parsley, rosemary, sage, savory, mint, tarragon, and thyme all add flavor to food. Purchase a culinary herb and spice book and learn how to use these seasonings.

Q. Are there any coffee substitutes?
A. My coffee-drinking friends say no. But Uncoffee, Pero, Cafix, and Postum are all grain drinks that make good substitutes. Herb teas can also take the place of coffee. To be satisfied

with a substitute you will need to program your mind away from coffee and toward better health.

Q. What about sea salt?
A. Sea salt is high in sodium. Herbs, spices, and mixed mineral salts make better seasonings.

ENERGY

Q. How can I increase my energy and stamina?
A. Eat a nutritious diet and take food supplements. Exercise at least three to five times a week. Get adequate sleep (seven to eight hours a night). If you try all the above and are still having problems, you may need to eat six small meals a day. If this doesn't help, take an attitude survey and see if you are worrying, harboring negative thoughts, or causing stress for yourself. Zig Ziglar calls this "stinking thinking," and it will steal your energy.

VITAMINS AND MINERALS

Q. Are vitamins and minerals toxic?
A. It depends on the amounts. Fat-soluble vitamins such as A, D, and E are stored in the liver and could become toxic in extremely high doses. *Megadoses* of minerals could be toxic as well since they can accumulate in the body. Minerals, however, sometimes have to be supplemented in low doses. Hair, urine, and blood analyses show these minerals: aluminum, lead, cadmium, mercury, and arsenic can reach extremely toxic levels and cause damage to the body.
  Some sources of these dangerous minerals are:

Aluminum—deodorants, aluminum foil, aluminum cookware, aluminum cans, antacids, and baking powder.
  Lead—automotive fumes, lead water pipes, hair dyes, contaminated food grown too close to highways.
  Cadmium—drinking water, cigarette smoke, refined foods, electroplating and decorative paints.
  Mercury—fish, insecticides, pesticides, and dental amalgams.

Arsenic—tobacco, pesticides, insecticides, defoliants.

The secret to keeping toxic minerals out of the cells is to make sure the cells contain nutritive minerals in the proper ratios.

Q. Are vitamin and mineral supplements necessary if we eat a balanced diet?

A. Pollution of our food and air makes it difficult to obtain totally unadulterated food, and our "hurry-up" lifestyle causes stress. Inadequate time spent on planning and food preparation and longtime storage of foodstuffs can result in an inadequate diet. If you live in a remote area, grow all your own food, keep the land minerally balanced, drink pure water, breathe pure air, and exercise daily, you probably won't need food supplements.

SCHOOL LUNCH

Q. What can be done about poor school lunches?

A. Pack a lunch for your child. Some schools are changing their lunch programs successfully to include nutritious lunches. For information about this write:
Sara Sloan Nutra
P. O. Box 13825
Atlanta, GA 30324

Q. How can we eliminate junk food sold at school?

A. Find some other interested parents and approach the school administrator to let you help organize selling apples, oranges, bananas, fruit juices, and yogurt. Then ask to have the candy and soft drink machines removed.

SLEEP

Q. What can help a person fall asleep faster?

A. Relaxing music, deep-breathing exercises, and prayer and meditation can help. Some find calcium or the amino acid tryptophan helps at bedtime.

WEIGHT LOSS

Q. What is the best way to control weight without all the ups and downs?

A. Dieting to lose weight must be a lifetime plan. A diabetic must follow a special diet forever, and an overweight person must do the same. Crash diets are rarely successful because eating patterns aren't changed. As soon as the weight is lost the old pattern reemerges, resulting in weight gain.

A medical checkup is essential before starting a diet. Then the body chemistry must be balanced. Food supplements may be necessary to bring this about. Calories must be figured and cut down. Junk food needs to be eliminated because of its "naked calories." Only nutritious food in small amounts should be eaten. Three to six *small* meals should be eaten daily. If you are hungry all the time, snack on low-calorie, high-fiber foods to fill your stomach. Also, aerobic exercise is essential to weight loss.

Each person is unique. What works for one may not work for another. Experiment and find what works best for you. Some people lose more on a high complex carbohydrate diet (beans, grains, fruits, and vegetables) and less protein. Others lose better on a higher protein diet and fewer carbohydrates. Most need to cut fat consumption to only small amounts. When you find something that works, stick with it.

Remember to eat slowly, chew your food thoroughly, drink water, and eat high-fiber foods to fill you up.

TESTS

Q. Are there any tests available to see what nutrients are low in my body?

A. Blood tests can be run to show the short-term nutrient levels present in the bloodstream. These levels fluctuate and are directly affected by food intake.

Urine is tested to help determine certain deficiencies.

Saliva can be tested in a limited way.

Hair is analyzed and will show the levels of minerals

present, as well as the levels of toxic minerals or metals hiding in the body. Minerals in the hair don't fluctuate daily. This is a more long-term measurement. Clinical symptoms and the patient's comments will often indicate a pattern to nutrient deficiencies. The clinician must listen to complaints of the patient to gather needed information.

Q. How can I get further education about mapping out my own preventative health plan?

A. Read and absorb the information in this book, and make a personal application of it. Consult books from the book list at the end of this chapter. Keep informed about current health information in magazines and newspapers. Exchange information with others. Attend health-related lectures and seminars when available. Purchase *Vita Charts* from Susanne Galloway, P.O. Box 2542, Prescott, AZ 86302. *The Nutrition Almanac* is available in bookstores. *Let's Live* magazine can be purchased from a health store or by subscription.

Q. What if I need additional nutritional advice?

A. Consult your medical doctor first. If he doesn't satisfy you, ask him to refer you to someone who can. There are nutritionists throughout the country. Ask doctors, dentists, psychologists, nurses, and your friends if they know a good nutritionist in your area.

Help me organize a winning team called "Do Something for Health." Based on what I hear and see around me, more and more people are concerned about *doing something*. The health of Americans can be improved if those who are aware of the problem do their part to help others learn to do their part.

When you finish reading this book, reread it. It is written not only to inform, but to motivate. I care about your health, and I want to help you. We have no guarantees about good health, for God alone is sovereign, but we are expected to care for the temple of the Holy Spirit. First Corinthians 6:19–20 instructs, "Do you not know that your body is a temple of the Holy Spirit who is in you, whom you have from God, and that you are not your own? For you have been bought with a price: therefore glorify God in your body" (NASB).

The first step toward good health is dependent upon our relationship to God. A warning is given in Matthew 16:26: "For what will a man be profited, if he gains the whole world, and forfeits his soul?" (NASB).

Jesus says in John 14:6, "I am the way, and the truth, and the life; no one comes to the Father, but through Me" (NASB). Everyone needs to make peace with God by receiving Jesus Christ as their personal Savior. He is life's never shifting foundation.

There are many steps built on top of the foundation for life. Carefully planned steps bring the most success.

As you think of your health, take a look at the steps toward good health contrasted to the steps toward failing health.

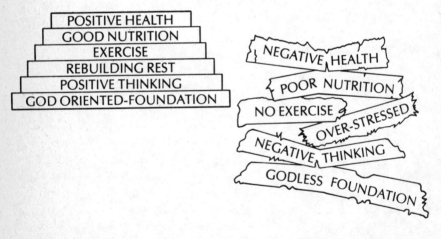

Fig 12.1 Winning Team vs. Losing Team. (Illustration by Louise Bauer)

Which is your choice? What team do you want to play on? Join the winning team.

Today is the day to start! Review your goals by turning back to chapter 11 and list them here again.

BLUEPRINT FOR HEALTH

1. _____

2. _____

3. _____

4. _____

5. _____

6. _____

As you start the race on the "Do Something for Health" team adopt the following motto to carry you through: "Whether, then, you eat or drink, or whatever you do, do all to the glory of God" (1 Corinthians 10:31 NASB).

SUGGESTED READING

All of the following suggested reading materials have educational merit. There are, however, a few areas in some of the books I would not wholeheartedly endorse. Read with discernment.

NUTRITIONAL BOOKS

Airola, Paavo. *How to Get Well*. Phoenix, Ariz: Health Plus Publishers, 1974.

Anderson, James W. *Diabetes: A Practical New Guide to Healthy Living*. New York: Arco Publishing, 1982.

Bieler, Henry G. *Food Is Your Best Medicine*. New York: Ballantine Books, 1982.

Brody, Jane. *Jane Brody's Nutrition Book*. New York: Bantam Books, 1982.

Cooper, Kenneth H. *Aerobics*. New York: Bantam Books, 1968.

Davis, Adelle. *Let's Eat Right to Keep Fit*. New York: Signet, New American Library, 1970.

———. *Let's Get Well*. New York: Harcourt, Brace & World, 1965.

Dong, Collin H., and Banks, Jane. *New Hope for the Arthritic*. New York: Ballantine Books, 1976.

Dufty, William. *Sugar Blues*. New York: Warner Books, 1975.

Eyton's, Audrey. *F-Plan Diet*. New York: Crown Publishers, 1982.

Feingold, Ben F. *Why Your Child Is Hyperactive*. New York: Random House, 1975.

Fredericks, Carlton, and Goodman, Herman. *Low Blood Sugar and You*. New York: Grosset and Dunlap, 1977.

Greenberg, Polly. *How to Convert the Kids From What They Eat to What They Oughta*. New York: Ballantine Books, 1980.

Hall, Ross Hume. *Food For Thought*. New York: Random House, 1974.

Holmes, Marjorie. *God and Vitamins*. Garden City, NY: Doubleday & Co., 1980.

Jacobson, Michael F. *Eater's Digest: The Consumer's Factbook of Food Additives*. Garden City, NY: Anchor Books, Doubleday & Co., 1976.

Kerschman, John D., Director. *Nutrition Almanac*. New York: McGraw-Hill Book Co., 1975.

Kline, Monte L., and Strube, W.P., Jr. *Eat, Drink and Be Ready*. Fort Worth, Tex.: Harvest Press, 1977.

Kuntzleman, Charles T. *Maximum Personal Energy*. Emmaus, Pa.: Rodale Press, 1981.

Lindberg, Gladys, and McFarland, Judy Lindberg. *Take Charge of Your Health*. San Francisco: Harper & Row, 1982.

Mendelsohn, Robert S. *Confessions of a Medical Heretic*. New York: Warner Books, 1980.

Pritikin, Nathan. *Pritikin Program for Diet and Exercise*. New York: Grosset and Dunlap, 1979.

Renwick, Ethel. *Let's Try Real Food*. Grand Rapids: Zondervan, 1982.

Rodale, J. I. *The Complete Book of Vitamins*. Emmaus, Pa.: Rodale Books, 1976.

————. *The Complete Book of Minerals for Health*. Emmaus, Pa.: Rodale Books, 1976.

Rohrer, Norman, and Rohrer, Virginia. *How to Eat Right and Feel Great*. Wheaton, Ill: Tyndale House Publishers, 1978.

Smith, Lendon. *Feed Your Kids Right*. New York: McGraw-Hill Book Co., 1979.

————. *Improving Your Child's Behavior Chemistry*. New York: Pocket Books, 1976.

Swope, Mary Ruth. *Nutrition For Christians*. Melbourne, Fla.: Swope Enterprises, 1981.

The Merck Manual. Rahway, N.J.: Merck, Sharp & Dohme Research Laboratories, 1977.

The Physicians Desk Reference. Oradell, N.J.: Medical Economics Co. / Charles E. Baker, Jr., 1980. (Drug listings, effects, side effects, and proper dosages.)

The Encyclopedia of Common Diseases. Edited by the Staff of *Prevention Magazine*. Emmaus, Pa.: Rodale Press, 1976.

Thurston, Emory W. *Nutrition for Tots to Teens*. Distributed by Institute of Nutritional Research. (Available from Susanne Galloway, P.O. Box 2542, Prescott, AZ 86302.)

Walker, Morton, and Gordon, Garry, M.D. *The Chelation Answer*. New York: M. Evans and Co., 1982.

Williams, Roger J. *Alcoholism: The Nutritional Approach*. Austin, Tex.: University of Texas Press, 1978.

————. *Nutrition Against Disease*. New York: Bantam Books, 1973.

————. *Nutrition in a Nutshell*. Garden City, NY: Dolphin Books, Doubleday & Co., 1962.

Yudkin, John. *Sweet and Dangerous*. New York: Bantam Books, 1972.

COOKBOOKS

A Collection of the Very Finest Recipes. Haywood, Ca: Cookbook Publishers.

Albright, Nancy. *The Rodale Cookbook*. Emmaus, Pa.: Rodale Press, 1973.

Emert, Judy. *Cookie Booklet, Cooking Naturally For Less, Natural Alternative*. Scottsdale, Ariz.: J.K. Enterprises. (Available from Susanne Galloway, P.O. Box 2542, Prescott, AZ 86302.)

Feingold, Ben F., and Feingold, Helen S. *The Feingold Cookbook For Hyperactive Children*. New York: Random House, 1979.

Goldbeck, David, and Goldbeck, Nikki. *The Good Breakfast Book*. New York: Links Books, 1976.

_____. *The Supermarket Handbook*. New York: Signet, New American Library, 1976.

Goodwin, Mary L., and Pollen, Gerry. *Creative Food Experiences For Children*. Washington: Center For Science in the Public Interest, 1980.

Hunter, Beatrice Trum. *The Natural Foods Cookbook*. New York: Harcourt Brace Jovanovich, 1976.

Kerr, Graham. *The Love Feast*. New York: Simon & Schuster, 1978.

Lappe, Frances Moore. *Diet for a Small Planet*. New York: Ballantine Books, 1975.

Larson, Gena, and Brown, Sam. *Fact Book for Better Babies and Their Families*. New Canaan, Conn.: Keats Publishing, 1972.

_____. *Cooking Creatively With Natural Foods*. New Canaan, Conn.: Keats Publishing.

Martin, Faye. *Naturally Delicious Desserts and Snacks*. Emmaus, Pa.: Rodale Press, 1978.

Renwick, Ethel. *The Real Food Cookbook*. Grand Rapids: Zondervan, 1978.

Thomas, Anna. *The Vegetarian Epicure*. New York: Alfred A. Knopf, 1972.

Thrash, Agatha M., M.D.. *Eat For Strength*. Seale, Ala.: Thrash Publications, 1983.

Thrash, Agatha Moody, M.D., and Thrash, Calvin L., Jr., M.D. *Nutrition for Vegetarians*. Seale, Ala.: Thrash Publications, 1982.

Turnbull, Yvonne. *The Living Cookbook*. Medford, Ore.: Omega Publishers, 1981.

Walker, N. W. *Diet and Salad Suggestions*. Phoenix, Ariz.: Norwalk Press, 1971.

SUGGESTED READING MATERIAL

Magazines and Newsletters

Let's Live—Los Angeles: Oxford Industries, Inc.

Bestways—Carson City, Nev.: Bestways Magazine, Inc.

Prevention—Emmaus, Pa.: Rodale Press, Inc.

Health Line
     The Robert A. McNeil Foundation
     2855 Campus Drive
     San Mateo, CA 94403

Nutrition Action
     Center for Science in the Public Interest
     1755 S. Street N.W.
     Washington, DC 20009

Health Facts
    Center for Medical Consumers
    237 Thompson Street
    New York, NY 10012
Federation of Homemakers, Inc.
    P.O. Box 5571
    Arlington, VA 22205
The Saturday Evening Post
    110 Waterway Boulevard
    Indianapolis, IN 46202

CHARTS
Vita Chart "Vitamins and Minerals" . . . Carolyn Heller West
    Susanne Galloway
    P.O. Box 2542
    Prescott, AZ 86302

Author's Address:
    Mary Ann Howard
    P.O. Box 2542
    Prescott, AZ 86302

NOTES

CHAPTER 2

[1]Clayton L. Thomas, *Taber's Cyclopedic Medical Dictionary*, 5th ed. (Philadelphia: F. A. Davis Co., 1975), F8.

[2]Institute of Medicine, *Healthy People: The Surgeon General's Report on Health Promotion and Disease Prevention* (Washington: U.S. Dept. of Health, Education and Welfare, U.S. Govt. Printing Office, 1979), vii-viii.

[3]*Senate Select Committee Report on Human Needs* (Washington: U.S. Govt. Printing Office, 1977).

[4]*Healthy People: The Surgeon General's Report*, 14.

[5]Ibid., 15.

[6]Ibid., 25.

CHAPTER 3

[1]Charles C. Ryrie, *Ryrie Study Bible*, NASB ED. (Chicago: Moody Press, 1976, 1978), 1540.

[2]Robert S. Mendelsohn, *Confessions of a Medical Heretic* (New York: Warner Books, 1980), 83.

[3]The *New York Times* (April 1979).

[4]Health and Science Research Committee Senate Hearing, 1978.

[5]Ibid.

[6]Marguerite Clark, *Medicine Today* (June 1960).

[7]Mary Ann Howard, *Christian Life* (June 1980): 38-40.

[8]Phyllis Lehmann, FDA Consumers Bulletin No. 81-3070 (Washington: U.S. Dept. of Health and Human Services, U.S. Govt. Printing Office, October 1981).

[9]Nutrition Foundation, *Present Knowledge in Nutrition* (Washington: Nutrition Foundation, 1984), 799, 806-9.

CHAPTER 4

[1]Carey Reams, "Water Consumption Formulas, Theory of Biological Ionization" (Phoenix: Class lecture, 25 April 1979).

[2]John Bartlett, *Familiar Quotations*, 13th ed. (Boston: Little, Brown, 1955), 21.

[3]Ibid.

CHAPTER 5

[1]Zig Ziglar, "I CAN" program for schools (Dallas: Zig Ziglar Corp.).

[2]Zig Ziglar (Prescott, Ariz.: Lecture, April 1980).

[3]Bartlett, *Familiar Quotations*, 323.

CHAPTER 6

[1]Catherine P. Anthony and Gary A. Thibodeau, *Textbook of Anatomy and Physiology,* 11th ed. (St. Louis: C. V. Mosby, 1983), 28. Used by permission.

[2]Mary E. Clark, *Contemporary Biology* (Philadelphia: W. B. Saunders, 1979), 110.

[3]Anthony and Thibodeau, *Textbook of Anatomy and Physiology,* 25. Used by permission.

[4]Ibid., 45. Used by permission.

[5]National Digestive Disease Advisory Board Report (Washington: U.S. Govt. Printing Office, 1979).

[6]Anthony and Thibodeau, *Textbook of Anatomy and Physiology,* 45. Used by permission.

[7]Ibid., 497-98. Used by permission.

[8]Ibid., 582. Used by permission.

[9]Adapted from Anthony and Thibodeau, *Textbook of Anatomy and Physiology,* 582.

CHAPTER 7

[1]Thomas, *Taber's Cyclopedic Medical Dictionary,* W2-3.

[2]*World Book Encyclopedia,* vol. 20 (Chicago: Field Enterprises Educational Corp., 1969), 95.

[3]The *Arizona Republic* (July 1978).

[4]The *Arizona Republic* (May 1982).

[5]Jane Brody, *Jane Brody's Nutrition Book* (New York: Bantam, 1982), 94-95.

[6]Ibid., 95.

[7]John Yudkin, *Sweet and Dangerous* (New York: Bantam, 1972), 100.

[8]Brody, *Jane Brody's Nutritional Book,* 126, 128.

[9]John D. Kirschmann, *Nutrition Almanac,* rev. ed. (New York: McGraw-Hill, 1975), 8.

[10]Nathan Pritikin, *Pritikin Program for Diet and Exercise* (New York: Grosset and Dunlap, 1979), 10-11.

[11]William Castelli, Framingham (Mass.) Heart Study.

[12]Samuel Epstein, *The Politics of Cancer* (San Francisco: Sierra Club Books, 1978), 439-40.

[13]Institute of Medicine, *Healthy People,* 129-30.

[14]Kirschmann, *Nutrition Almanac,* 9.

[15]Thomas, *Taber's Cyclopedic Medical Dictionary,* U8.

[16]*Nutritive Value of American Foods, Agriculture Handbook No. 456 (Washington: U.S. Govt. Printing Office, 1979).*

[17]Ibid.

[18]Food and Nutrition Board of the National Academy of Sciences.

CHAPTER 8

[1]Associated Press: quoted by John Goodwin, The *Arizona Republic*, (25 August 1983).

[2]Thomas, *Taber's Cyclopedic Medical Dictionary*, V27-29.

[3]J. I. Rodale, *The Complete Book of Vitamins (Emmaus, Pa.: Rodale Books, 1976), 13.*

[4]Ibid.

[5]Kirschmann, *Nutrition Almanac*, 196.

[6]Thomas, *Taber's Cyclopedic Medical Dictionary*, A147.

[7]Wilfred E. Shute, *The Vitamin E Book* (New Canaan, Conn.: Keats Publishing, 1978), 59-61.

[8]Thomas, *Taber's Cyclopedic Medical Dictionary*, V29.

[9]Shute, *The Vitamin E Book, 45-46.*

[10]J. I. Rodale, *The Complete Book of Minerals* (Emmaus, Pa.: Rodale Books, 1976), xv.

[11]Thomas, *Taber's Cyclopedic Medical Dictionary*, M53.

[12]Rodale, *The Complete Book of Minerals*, xvii–xviii.

[13]Ibid., xvi.

[14]Kirschmann, *Nutrition Almanac*, 196-98.

[15]Carolyn Heller West, *Vita Chart* (New York: Vita Chart, 1982).

[16]Thomas, *Taber's Cyclopedic Medical Dictionary*, E43, E45.

[17]Max Wolf and Karl Ransberger, *Enzyme Therapy* (Los Angeles: Regent House, 1977), 13.

[18]H. C. Biddle and V. W. Foutz, *Chemistry in Health and Disease,* 6th ed. (Philadelphia: F. A. Davis Co., 1965): Quoted in Thomas, *Taber's Cyclopedic Medical Dictionary*, E43.

[19]Thomas, *Taber's Cyclopedic Medical Dictionary*, E44.

[20]David Reuben, *The Save Your Life Diet* (New York: Random House, 1975), xii.

[21]Ibid., 7.

[22]Brody, *Jane Brody's Nutrition Book*, 144.

[23]James W. Anderson, *Diabetes* (New York: Arco Publishing, 1981), 141-43.

[24]Ibid., 112.

[25]Ibid., 127.

[26]Ibid., 141-42.

CHAPTER 9

[1]Clark, *Contemporary Biology*, 7.

[2]Ibid., 12.

[3]*Nutrition in Action* (Washington: Center for Science in the Public Interest, October 1983).

[4]Ibid., 3.

[5]Reams, Class lecture.

[6]Ross Hume Hall, *Food for Nought* (New York: Harper & Row, 1974), 20-21.

[7]Institute of Medicine, *Healthy People.*

[8]Henry G. Beiler, *Food Is Your Best Medicine* (New York: Ballantine, 1982), 189.

[9]Michael F. Jacobson, "Chemical Cuisine Information Chart," adapted from *Eater's Digest* (Garden City, N.J.: Doubleday, Anchor Books, 1976).

[10]Michael F. Jacobson, *Eater's Digest* (Garden City, N.J.: Doubleday, Anchor, 1976), app. 1.

[11]Monte Kline and W. P. Strube, Jr., *Eat, Drink, and Be Ready* (Fort Worth: Harvest Press, 1977), 174.

CHAPTER 10

[1]Weston A. Price, *Nutrition and Physical Degeneration* (Santa Monica: Price-Pottenger Nutrition Foundation, 1977), 187. Used by permission, the Price-Pottenger Nutrition Foundation, P.O. Box 2614, La Mesa, CA 92041.

[2]Ibid., 196.

[3]Ibid., 198.

[4]Ibid., 200.

[5]Marion Mason et al., *Nutrition and the Cell: The Inside Story* (Chicago: Yearbook Medical Publishers, 1973), 121.

[6]Elie Shneour, *The Malnourished Mind* (Garden City, N.J.: Doubleday, Anchor, 1974).

[7]Roger J. Williams, *Nutrition Against Disease* (New York: Pittman Publishing, 1971), 34.

[8]Collin Dong and Jane Banks, *New Hope for the Arthritic* (New York: Ballantine, 1976), 2-4. Used by permission.

[9]Ibid., 34-36. Used by permission.

CHAPTER 11

[1]David L. Messenger, *Dr. Messenger's Guide to Better Health* (Old Tappan, N.J.: Fleming H. Revell, 1981), 116-17.

[2]Norman Cousins, *Dr. Schweitzer of Lamberene* (New York: Harper & Row, 1960).

[3]Norman Cousins, *Anatomy of an Illness* (New York: W. W. Norton, 1979), 39-40.

[4]Ibid., 32.

[5]Institute of Medicine, *Healthy People,* 62.

[6]Ibid., 67.

[7]Charles T. Kuntzleman, *Maximum Personal Energy* (Emmaus, Pa.: Rodale Press, 1981), 88.

[8]Ibid., 89.

[9]Ibid., 92.

[10]Ibid., 103.

[11]Kenneth Cooper, *Aerobics* (New York: M. Evans, 1968), 22.

[12]Ibid., 15.

[13]Hans Selye, *Stress Without Distress* (New York: Harper & Row, 1974), 34.

[14]"About Laxatives and B.M.s," *Executive Health Newsletter,* vol. 8, no. 11.

CHAPTER 12

[1]Arthur F. Coco, *The Pulse Test* (New York: Arco Publishing, 1978).

[2]Roger J. Williams, *Alcoholism, the Nutritional Approach* (Austin: University of Texas Press, 1978), 93-94.

[3]Ibid., 86.

[4]Ibid., 87.

[5]Morton Walker and Garry Gordon, *The Chelation Answer* (New York: M. Evans, 1982), 14.

[6]Polly Greenberg, *How to Convert the Kids From What They Eat to What They Oughta* (New York: Ballantine, 1978), 4.

INDEX

Isoleucine 62

Jacobson, Michael 97, 100, 146
Jane Brody's Nutrition Book 146
Junk food 13-14, 35, 41, 141-42

Kellogg, John Harvey 87, 106-8
Kidneys 29, 44, 47, 53, 55, 62, 74, 135
Kline, Monte 146

Lappe, Frances Moore 148
Laxative 130-31
Lecithin 72
Legumes 61-62, 68, 71-72, 79-81, 94, 131
Lentils 37, 39, 65, 87, 91, 118
Leucine 62
Lipase 85
Liver: as food 25, 64, 70-73, 75, 79-81; organ 16, 29, 37, 47-48, 74, 99, 123-24, 128-29, 140
Longevity Center 58
Lunch 13-14, 17, 30, 99, 120, 141
Lysine 62, 137

Magnesium 62, 75, 79, 82, 88, 125, 128, 134
Malnourished Personal Energy 124-25, 146
Manganese 79, 81, 83
Margarine 76, 81
Meals 9-10, 14, 17, 30, 39, 75, 97, 109, 116, 119, 128, 140, 142; charts 109-118
Meat 9, 13, 17, 36-37, 58, 65, 70-72, 76, 80-81, 87, 97, 115, 138
Mendelsohn, Robert S. 19, 147
Messenger, David 122
Metabolism 40, 63, 69, 83
Methionine 61-62
Milk 25, 58, 61-62, 65-66, 68, 71-73, 76, 79-81, 97, 99, 118, 125, 130-31, 135, 139

Minerals 27, 38, 53, 62, 68-69, 76-77, 79, 82, 84, 95, 101, 106, 115, 128-29, 134, 140, 142, 147, 149; chart 79-81
Molasses 71-73, 79-81
Monosodium glutamate (MSG) 134
Muscles 40, 42, 52, 61, 82, 125

National Digestive Disease Advisory Board 45
Nervous system 42, 124-25
New Hope for the Arthritic 119, 146
New York Times 19
Niacin 70, 72, 109
Nutrients 11-12, 44, 52, 56, 71, 74, 76, 83, 94, 106, 108, 119, 123, 128, 130, 138, 142
Nutrition Almanac 143, 146
Nutrition Against Disease 147
Nutrition and Physical Degeneration 103
Nutrition "thieves" 105-6, 108
Nuts 9, 23, 32, 68, 71-73, 80-81, 87, 9, 103, 107, 111, 119, 130

Oatmeal 65, 73, 87, 106-7, 109, 118
Obesity 56, 83, 87-88, 106
Oils 58, 73, 76
Orange juice 80, 99, 106
Organ meats 58, 71-73, 80-81
Osteoporosis 82

Pangamic acid 70, 72
Pantothenic acid 70, 72, 76, 128
Pasta 14
Peanut butter 58, 65, 80, 107, 111
Peanuts 58, 61, 72
Peas 37, 39, 61, 66, 69, 75, 80, 87, 91, 110, 115, 118
Pecans 58, 118
Pesticides 59, 93, 141
Phenylalanine 62
Phosphorus 62, 80, 88

BLUEPRINT FOR HEALTH